# CSA 3rd EDITION

# SCENARIOS FOR THE

# MRCGP

Health Library
Clinical Education Centre
University Hospitals of North Midlands Trust
Royal Stoke University Hospital
Newcastle Road
Stoke-on-Trent
ST4 6QG

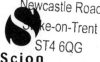

Scion

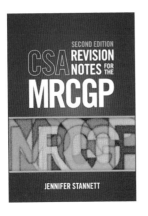
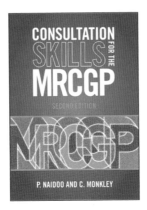
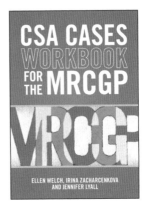
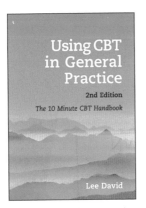
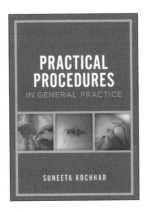
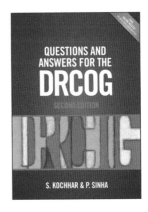
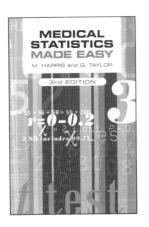
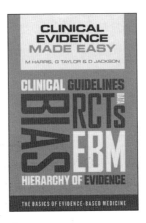
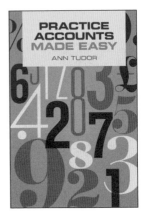

# CSA
## 3rd EDITION
## SCENARIOS FOR THE
# MRCGP

### FRAMEWORKS FOR CLINICAL CONSULTATIONS

**THOMAS M. DAS**
MBBS, MRCGP, DCH, BSc (Hons)
GP in London

Scion

© **Scion Publishing Limited, 2015**

ISBN 978 1 907904 63 9

Third edition first published 2015

Second edition published 2011, reprinted 2012, 2013, 2014

First edition published 2009, reprinted 2010, 2011

**Scion Publishing Limited**

The Old Hayloft, Vantage Business Park, Bloxham Road, Banbury OX16 9UX, UK

www.scionpublishing.com

**Important Note from the Publisher**

The information contained within this book was obtained by Scion Publishing Ltd from sources believed by us to be reliable. However, while every effort has been made to ensure its accuracy, no responsibility for loss or injury whatsoever occasioned to any person acting or refraining from action as a result of information contained herein can be accepted by the authors or publishers.

Readers are reminded that medicine is a constantly evolving science and while the authors and publishers have ensured that all dosages, applications and practices are based on current  indications, there may be specific practices which differ between communities. You should always follow the guidelines laid down by the manufacturers of specific products and the relevant authorities in the country in which you are practising.

Although every effort has been made to ensure that all owners of copyright material have been acknowledged in this publication, we would be pleased to acknowledge in subsequent reprints or editions any omissions brought to our attention.

Registered names, trademarks, etc. used in this book, even when not marked as such, are not to be considered unprotected by law.

Typeset by Phoenix Photosetting, Chatham, Kent, UK

Printed in the UK

# Contents

## Section 1 – An approach to the CSA

## Section 2 – Special GP cases

## Section 3 – Typical cases

### Cardiovascular

## Respiratory

## Gastro-intestinal

## Endocrinology

## Musculo-skeletal

# Neurology

# Dermatology

# ENT

# Ophthalmology

# Genito-urinary and men's health

# Sexual health

# Renal

# Women's health

# Paediatrics

# Psychiatry

# Appendices

# Guideline summaries

# Preface to the third edition

This new updated edition is the result of countless hours of navigating through the latest clinical evidence, national guidelines, and medical literature, so that you can concentrate your efforts on passing the CSA exam itself.

I am delighted that the previous editions have helped thousands of candidates in their exam preparation since it was first published six years ago. I have therefore tried to keep to the original's vision of creating a concise "need-to-know" guide to passing the CSA, with the emphasis on successfully completing a case in the allotted 10 minutes using a structured consultation framework that works.

The existing cases have been updated and new topics added. Where appropriate I have added summaries of national guidelines to further supplement the cases.

Section 1 has been reworked to reflect current practice and encourage the reader to build upon their own consultation style. As with the rest of life, we must use what works for us and build upon the skills and knowledge we already possess.

I wish you every success, both in the CSA and beyond!

**Thomas M. Das**
August 2014

# Preface to the second edition

This book is based upon the set of notes I compiled and used to pass the Clinical Skills Assessment (CSA) part of the new MRCGP. In the following pages over 100 cases are presented in a structured format optimised for exam success.

I found that the real difficulty was not only gathering vast amounts of information from up-to-date sources into a consultation structure, but also to distil it so the case can be completed in 10 minutes.

Therefore this book aims to:
1. provide up-to-date information in a concise, structured and accessible manner
2. enable the candidate to complete the case in 10 minutes

While this book is not a comprehensive textbook of medicine, I have included summaries of certain "hot topics" where appropriate.

So use the cases, make sure you see plenty of real patients and practise, practise, practise.

Good luck!

**Thomas M. Das**
August 2008

## Acknowledgements

Thank you to Shiv Shanmugaratnam, Robin Clark, Jonathan Behr, Serena Foo, and Aisha Laskor for your helpful comments and feedback.

Thank you to my dad for giving me the opportunity to study medicine.

The biggest thanks go to my wife Thao and my two beautiful sons Leo and Joshua for their support and much welcome distraction respectively, both of which have been invaluable in writing this third edition.

## Dedication

I dedicate this book to my mum and her mum for their bravery and love, and for encouraging me to always follow my heart. Thank you.

# Abbreviations

| | | | |
|---|---|---|---|
| AAA | Abdominal aortic aneurysm | FEV1 | Forced expiratory volume in 1 second |
| A&E | Accident and emergency department | FSH | Follicle stimulating hormone |
| ABPM | Ambulatory blood pressure monitoring | FVC | Forced vital capacity |
| | | GABHS | Group A beta-haemolytic *Streptococci* |
| ACEi | ACE inhibitor | | |
| ACR | Albumin–creatinine ratio | GCS | Glasgow Coma Scale |
| ACS | Acute coronary syndrome | GFR | Glomerular filtration rate |
| ADL | Activities of daily living | GI | Gastro-intestinal |
| AF | Atrial fibrillation | GMC | General Medical Council |
| ARB | Angiotensin receptor blocker | GORD | Gastro-oesophageal reflux disease |
| dBP | Diastolic blood pressure | | |
| sBP | Systolic blood pressure | GPCOG | General practitioner assessment of cognition |
| BMI | Body mass index | | |
| BP | Blood pressure | GTN | Glyceryl trinitrate |
| BPAD | Bipolar affective disorder | GU | Genito-urinary |
| CBT | Cognitive behavioural therapy | GUM | Genito-urinary medicine |
| CCB | Calcium channel blocker | Hb | Haemoglobin |
| CCF | Congestive cardiac failure | HBPM | Home blood pressure monitoring |
| CHD | Chronic heart disease | | |
| CI | Contraindication | HTN | Hypertension |
| CKD | Chronic kidney disease | I&D | Incision and drainage |
| CKS | Clinical Knowledge Summaries | IBD | Inflammatory bowel disease |
| COCP | Combined oral contraceptive pill | IBS | Irritable bowel syndrome |
| COPD | Chronic obstructive pulmonary disease | ICE | Ideas, concerns and expectations |
| | | ICS | Inhaled corticosteroid |
| CRF | Chronic renal failure | IDA | Iron deficient anaemia |
| CRP | C-reactive protein | IMB | Inter-menstrual bleeding |
| CSA | Clinical skills assessment | IPT | Interpersonal therapy |
| CSF | Cerebro-spinal fluid | IUD | Intrauterine device (e.g. copper coil) |
| CVD | Cardiovascular disease | | |
| CVS | Cardiovascular system | IUS | Intrauterine system (e.g. Mirena) |
| CXR | Chest X-ray | | |
| DH | Drug history | IVDU | Intravenous drug user |
| DM | Diabetes mellitus | LA | Local anaesthetic |
| DMARD | Disease-modifying antirheumatic drug | LFTs | Liver function tests |
| | | LMP | Last menstrual period |
| DRE | Digital rectal exam | LOC | Loss of consciousness |
| DSH | Deliberate self harm | LRTI | Lower respiratory tract infection |
| DVLA | Driver and Vehicle Licensing Agency | LTOT | Long-term oxygen therapy |
| | | MAOIs | Monoamine oxidase inhibitors |
| DVT | Deep vein thrombosis | MCS | Microscopy, culture and sensitivities |
| E&D | Eating and drinking | | |
| ECG | Electrocardiogram | MDT | Multidisciplinary team |
| ESR | Erythrocyte sedimentation rate | MSU | Mid-stream urine |
| FBC | Full blood count | | |

| | | | |
|---|---|---|---|
| NAI | Non-accidental injury | RA | Rheumatoid arthritis |
| NICE | National Institute for Health and Care Excellence | RhF | Rheumatoid factor |
| | | RICE | Rest, ice, compression, elevation |
| NIV | Non-invasive ventilation | | |
| NRT | Nicotine replacement therapy | RR | Respiratory rate |
| NSAID | Non-steroidal anti-inflammatory drug | RVF | Right ventricular failure |
| | | Rx | Treatment |
| NTDs | Neural tube defects | SE | Side effect |
| OA | Osteoarthritis | SIGN | Scottish Intercollegiate Guidelines Network |
| OCP | Ova, cysts and parasites | | |
| OGTT | Oral glucose tolerance test | SOB | Shortness of breath |
| ORS | Oral rehydration salt (solution) | SSRI | Selective serotonin reuptake inhibitor |
| OSA | Obstructive sleep apnoea | | |
| OTC | Over-the-counter | STI | Sexually transmitted infection |
| PCB | Post-coital bleeding | Sz | Schizophrenia |
| PE | Pulmonary embolism | T2DM | Type 2 diabetes mellitus |
| PEFR | Peak expiratory flow rate | TATT | Tired all the time |
| PID | Pelvic inflammatory disease | TCA | Tricyclic antidepressant |
| PND | Paroxysmal nocturnal dyspnoea | TFTs | Thyroid function tests |
| PO | *Per orum* | TIA | Transient ischaemic attack |
| POP | Progesterone only contraceptive pill | TOP | Termination of pregnancy |
| | | U&Es | Urea and electrolytes |
| PPI | Proton pump inhibitor | UPSI | Unprotected sexual intercourse |
| PR | *Per rectum* | URTI | Upper respiratory tract infection |
| PTSD | Post-traumatic stress disorder | USS | Ultrasound scan |
| PVD | Peripheral vascular disease | VTE | Venous thrombo-embolism |

# How to use this book

This book has primarily been written to help you to succeed in passing the CSA part of the MRCGP examination. I have therefore kept the text concise and suggestions directive and practical. The following pages outline various strategies, tips and frameworks that have helped me and thousands of other candidates pass the CSA exam, and continue to help me today in my practice as a GP.

The first section suggests a practical approach to the CSA which is appropriate for a 10 minute GP consultation as well as fulfilling the marking criteria of the MRCGP. Whilst the CSA has both its advantages and disadvantages as an examination, one of its great assets is its weighting on interpersonal skills. This means that in striving to pass the CSA exam you are also striving to conduct an efficient and *patient-centred* consultation – one which explores the patient's feelings and addresses his or her concerns, and so one that responds to a person and not just a symptom. To this end I have provided ideas and suggested specific phrases that can be used in the 10 minute consultation. Relationships, however, are not something that can be reduced to a simple formula or tick box, and the doctor–patient relationship is no different. Every doctor has their own unique consultation style and I would advise you to experiment, incorporating the suggestions that work for you.

The second section addresses more "real life" GP consultations that often do not fit into a standard medical model of disease. I have provided alternative suggested approaches to these cases, incorporating national guidance where available.

The third section identifies symptoms and conditions that you may face in the exam, suggesting a framework through which you can approach the case. One of the problems GP trainees have to face is the huge breadth of knowledge required to be a GP. This challenge is taken one step further in the CSA as the candidate must demonstrate effective use of this information within a 10 minute consultation. I have searched through the latest evidence and guidelines to provide you with a set of comprehensive notes detailing what you need to know.

# Section 1
# An approach to the CSA

# How to pass the CSA – full marks in 10 minutes

Each case is marked using three equally weighted domains:
1. data gathering
2. management
3. interpersonal skills

The key is to complete all of the above domains for all cases competently within the allocated 10 minutes. Here are the five key steps needed to do this.

---

**The five key steps**
1. Initial open question
2. Targeted history with red flags/examination
3. Ideas, concerns, expectations (ICE) and effect on day-to-day life
4. Explain diagnosis and shared management plan
5. Safety net/arrange follow up

---

Keeping to this basic structure will ensure all domains are covered. The red flags and safety net ensure the consultation is safe. Many candidates swap steps 2 and 3 around, so ICE is asked earlier on, and this can often be a good way of eliciting a patient-centred history.

All five steps pose a challenge to the CSA candidate, but most find steps 2 and 4 especially difficult. Therefore while this book covers all five steps, it goes into more detail on steps 2 and 4.

---

**During the exam**
Writing down the five key steps on the notepaper provided in the exam will prompt you to cover all three domains regardless of your nerves

---

Interpersonal skills will be demonstrated throughout the 10 minutes.

Each step, together with interpersonal skills will be expanded in the next sections.

It is important to verbalise what you are thinking in the exam. You cannot obtain marks for unspoken thoughts, for example, if you are concerned about patient's safety at home or are unsure if they understand what is being said. Similarly, if you offer to give written information, you will only gain marks if you have explained the contents of written materials.

# Basic consultation structure

This section expands on the five key steps outlined in the previous section.

## 1. Initial open question

*"Hello, my name is Dr X... What brings you here today?"*

Then actively listen: make eye contact, gently smile and nod whilst listening.

The actor will volunteer a set amount of information. In some cases, this will purposely not be very much. Follow up with a second open question you already have up your sleeve:

*"Could you tell me more about ................?"*

Very occasionally a third open question will be needed; try:

*"How did it all begin?"*

---

**Initial open questions**

These three simple open questions can be lifesavers during the CSA:
1. *"What brings you here today?"*
2. *"Can you tell me more about ................?"*
3. *"How did it all begin?"*

---

## 2. Targeted history with red flags/examination

Try to cover all the main headings in the table below for each case. Often most of the information will already be covered in the patient summary sheet. However, it is possible that not all relevant information will be given, reflecting real life.

| Targeted history | Key questions |
|---|---|
| Presenting complaint | *"What do you mean by 'migraine'?"* |
| History | *"Have you ever had this before?"* <br> *"Have you already tried anything?"* <br> *"Was there anything in particular that made you to come to see a doctor now (rather than before)?"* |
| Past medical history, family history, and drug history | Drug concordance, OTC/herbal remedies |

| Targeted history | Key questions |
|---|---|
| Social history | |
|     Home/work/relationships | "Who lives at home?" |
|     Smoking/alcohol/recreational drugs | "How are things at work? Outside work?" |
|     Driving | "Has anything happened at home/work?" |
| Red flags | Weight loss |
| | Bleeding (PO/PV/PR/GU) |
| | Pain (chest, bone, ...) |

---

**During the exam – red flags**

Red flags are specific to the condition, but a simple rule is to ask about:

1. weight loss
2. bleeding
3. pain

---

Examine for red flags and specific signs only if case requires – see later chapters for more information on this.

# 3. ICE and effect on life

There are four main questions (I, C, E and effect on life; see box below). It is important to ask these questions using a warm and caring tone of voice. It can be especially useful to ask the questions slowly, even hesitantly, thus demonstrating your concern and sensitivity to the patient.

---

**ICE (ideas, concerns, expectations)**

"Do you have any idea what is causing this?"

"Is there anything in particular that you are concerned about?"

"Is there anything in particular you were hoping I could do for you today?"

**Effect on life**

"How does this affect your day-to-day life?"

   or

"Does it stop you from doing anything?"

An alternative is:

"How are you coping with/finding it all?"

---

For most cases, it is important to ensure that all these four questions are asked at some point. When to ask which question will vary depending upon the presenting complaint. You may find that you prefer to ask about ICE much earlier on, e.g. immediately after your initial open question(s), and many candidates find this a useful way to elicit a history and get to the nub of the consultation. This is especially true for psychiatric and social-type cases, but also true for many physical health symptoms.

ICE can also be used if you are stuck (see also *"What to do if your mind goes blank"* section below).

At this point it can also be useful to summarise the history to the patient. This not only shows that you have been actively listening, but ensures you have not missed anything out and gives the patient a chance to correct any wrong information.

# 4. Explain diagnosis and shared management plan

This step is one of the most difficult parts of the CSA. The approach will vary depending on the type of case, but here are some suggested guidelines. Specific pointers are given within each case in Sections 2 and 3 of this book.

*Use jargon free language*
Try to use the same words as the patient if possible. The specific cases in *Sections 2* and *3* provide advice on this. Practising with a non-medic is also useful here.

*Tell the patient your diagnosis*
Or tell them of the possible diagnoses or simply your understanding of their situation.

Check their understanding of this (i.e. their *ideas*).

*Give management options*
Often there will be more than one option, but sometimes it will be necessary to recommend urgent management (e.g. if the patient has red flags). Give rationale for investigations and treatments where appropriate, especially if urgent management is needed.

*Involve the patient in the "shared management plan"*
Address the patient's ideas, concerns and expectations (ICE) as well as the effect on the patient's day-to-day life.

Ask the patient what they think of the diagnosis and management plan. Check the patient's understanding, e.g. do they already have an idea of what the treatment options are?

If you are breaking bad news, see *Section 2*.

*Possible investigations*
These can generally be divided into three areas: *bedside*, *bloods*, and *imaging*.

| Bedside | Urine dip and MCS, infection swab, sputum |
|---|---|
| Blood tests | FBC, U&Es, ... |
| Imaging | CXR, ultrasound, ECG |

*Management options*
These can generally be divided into three areas: *conservative*, *medical*, and *surgical*.

| Conservative<br>• specific<br>• social<br>• lifestyle | Wait and see<br>Physiotherapy, relaxation exercises, psychology<br>Inform DVLA, sick note<br>Weight loss, smoking cessation, alcohol reduction, healthy diet, exercise |
|---|---|
| Medical | Analgesia, PPI, antihypertensives |
| Surgical | Joint injections, minor and major surgery |

Throughout the cases in this book, the various investigations listed are merely *suggested investigations*. The appropriateness of which investigation to use or whether to investigate at all are all specific to the individual case.

# 5. Safety net and arrange follow up

Tell patient when to seek help, e.g. if not improving in 4–6 weeks, if concerned or red flags. Arrange follow up either with yourself or another health care professional (e.g. nurse, specialist). Refer if appropriate.

# Consultation structure – summary

## The five key steps

1. Initial open question
2. Targeted history with red flags
3. Ideas, concerns, expectations (ICE) and effect on day-to-day life
4. Explain diagnosis and shared management plan
5. Safety net/arrange follow up

## Data gathering

*Introduction*   Open question(s)
  *"What brings you here today?"*
  *"Can you tell me more about 'X'?"*
  *"How did it all begin?"*

*Targeted history*   Presenting complaint
  *"What do you mean by 'X'?"*
  *"Have you ever had this before?"*
  *"Have you already tried anything?"*
  *"Was there anything in particular that made you come to see a doctor now (rather than before)?"*
  Past medical history
  Family history
  Drug history
  Drug concordance, OTC/herbal remedies

*Social history*   Home, job, relationships
  *"Who lives at home?"*
  *"How are things at work? Outside work?"*
  *"Has anything happened at home/work?"*
  Smoking, alcohol, drugs

*Red flags*   e.g. bleeding, pain, weight loss
  Examination if required

*Targeted examination*   If required

## Interpersonal skills

*ICE and effect*
*on daily life*
"*Do you have any idea what is causing this?*"
"*Is there anything in particular that you are concerned about?*"
"*Is there anything in particular you were hoping I could do for you today?*"
"*How does this affect your day-to-day life?*" and/or "*Does it stop you from doing anything?*"
"*How are you coping with it all?*"
Summarise history

*For patient*  Explain diagnosis

## Management

*Suggested*
*investigations*
Urine, bloods, imaging if required

*Management*
*options*
Conservative, medical, surgical
Lifestyle, social

*Safety net*  Arrange follow up
Consider referral (e.g. if red flags)

# Interpersonal skills

Whole books have been written on consultation skills, but in-depth knowledge of the various models is not required to pass the CSA. Here are some straightforward practical pointers to get you through (see also *Appendix: Suggested phrases during a consultation*). Practising with a non-medic is also useful here.

## General pointers to build rapport

*Non-verbal*: eye contact, smile.

*Verbal*: speak clearly, soft tone of voice, avoid monotonous tone/vary pitch of voice.

*Active listening*: gently nodding head, open body language, non-judgemental.

## Pick up cues

If the patient mentions a specific point, appears upset/anxious, etc., you can comment on these 'cues'. This not only builds rapport, but can also open the consultation and provide you with new information. Don't forget to pause and allow the patient time to respond.

Here are some phrases you can use as a response to non-verbal cues from the patient:

> *"How are you feeling?"*
> *"How do you feel about what's been said so far?"*
> *"I can see that you're upset by that…"*

Note, for the last suggestion you should only label a non-verbal cue if you are sure the patient is feeling a certain way – otherwise you risk a response such as "No, I'm not upset!". If a patient appears uncomfortable/anxious/upset but you are not sure, it is much better simply to question how they are feeling).

Here is an example of how you could respond to a verbal cue from a patient:

> *"You mentioned you look after your grandmother…"*

## Empathy and 'empathy statements'

It is important to be able to demonstrate your emotional understanding of what the patient is going through. For the exam it is important that you have some phrases you feel comfortable and natural with. Here are a few suggested "empathy statements". After each sentence, don't forget to pause, as this allows the patient some breathing space and perhaps they may open up further.

- *"That must be very difficult for you..."*
- *"Sounds like you've been through a lot..."*
- *"I'm so sorry to hear that..."*
- *"I understand that must be quite annoying for you..."*

## Difficult, direct or intrusive questions and consultations

As doctors we sometimes have to ask difficult questions, e.g. when suspecting domestic violence, child maltreatment or suicidal ideation. Other situations include dealing with sensitive information, such as when breaking bad news, during TOP counselling, or even asking why a patient did not obtain treatment previously (with the intent of not making them feel guilty or foolish).

I have found that even the most direct of questions can be asked if spoken in a <u>soft and caring tone with a slow and almost hesitant pace</u>. It's not only what you say, but how you say it. Exactly how you incorporate this will vary on your own consultation style, so experiment and find out the vocal tone and pace that work best for you.

## Social context of symptoms

- ICE – address patient's ideas, concerns and expectations.
- Contextualise the symptoms in terms of the patient's life: work, home, relationships.
- Remain non-judgemental and sympathetic.

# What if your mind goes blank?

This is an area that I often found myself suffering from, with my mind going blank mid-consultation.

There are several strategies, as set out below.

## 1. Practise by role-playing and with patients

This is essential. The more you practise cases with colleagues and with real patients, the less your mind will go blank – the book *Consultation Skills for the new MRCGP* by Prashini Naidoo will help with this.

## 2. Open questions

This strategy is more useful at the beginning of the consultation. Remember the three initial open questions and ICE/effect on life:

*"Could you tell me more about this?"*

*"How did it all begin?"*

*"Do you have any ideas what could be causing this?"* (ICE)

## 3. Summarise

This strategy is more useful if you get stuck during history taking. Tell the patient what you know so far. The process of going through this out loud is often enough to jolt your mind back into being the history taking machine that you already are.

## 4. Use the five key steps

Here's where it can be useful to note the five key steps at the beginning of the CSA when you are arranging your equipment (see box below).

## 5. Go through the history

Ensure you have covered history of the presenting complaint, past medical history, family history, drug history, social history (including work, home, smoking, alcohol, driving).

People often forget family history, driving, and effect on life. How relevant these are will vary from case to case.

For pain, use SOCRATES (site, onset, character, radiation, alleviating factors, time course, exacerbating factors, severity).

**During the exam**

Write down the following two lists on a blank piece of paper just before the exam. A quick glance at this when you are stuck will get you going again.

*List 1: The History*
- History of presenting complaint (HPC)
- Past medical history (PMH)
- Drug history (DH)
- Family history (FH)
- Social history (SH)

*List 2: The 5 Key Steps*
- History
- Red flags (includes examination if required)
- Diagnosis
- Investigations and management
- Follow up

# Section 2
# Special GP cases

# Telephone consultation

This can be approached as a normal consultation, but with the emphasis shifted to obtaining enough information over the telephone to determine what the action plan should be and ensuring that adequate safety-netting is in place.

Key considerations during a telephone consultation:
- Is the person you are talking to the patient? Try to talk to the patient directly where possible.
- If they are not the patient is there an issue of confidentiality? Are they correctly communicating the patient's symptoms and medical history? Are they an adult?
- ICE, as ever, is important to ascertain early on in the consultation.
- Could the patient be depressed or anxious? This can easily be missed in the absence of visual cues and the patient may prefer not to see someone in person.
- What is the patient wanting from the telephone consultation, e.g. are they looking for telephone advice, a blood test, emotional support, a home visit or a GP appointment?
- Does the patient need to come in for a face-to-face assessment? If so, when (today, tomorrow, next week)? Are they able to travel?
- If the patient does not need to come in to see you, do they have enough support at home?

## Data gathering

| | |
|---|---|
| *Preparation* | Familiarise yourself with patient's relevant clinical details |
| *Introduce yourself* | *"Hello, my name is Dr X, a GP from Y Medical Centre"* |
| *Confirms patient's identity* | *"I understand you wanted to speak to a doctor today?"* <br> *"Yes that's right"* <br> *"Before we proceed could you please confirm your name and date of birth?"* |
| *Open question(s)* | *"How can I help today?"* |
| *Targeted history* | Include targeted systems review (see Appendix 2) |
| *Social history* | As appropriate |
| *Red flags* | Especially important to ask about these given lack of visual cues |

# Interpersonal skills

*ICE and effect*   Warm tone of voice is important to establish rapport
*on daily life*   Be sensitive to patient's mood and don't be afraid to ask how they are
      feeling or if their symptoms are getting them down.
    ICE early on to understand what is worrying the patient and what they are
      expecting from you
    Allow patient time to ask questions and voice concerns
    Summarise / repeat advice
    Ask patient to repeat back information to check they have correctly
      understood
    Ensure all patient's concerns have been addressed before ending phone call

# Management

*Investigations*   As necessary

*Management*   Options include:
    Telephone advice +/– online information leaflets
    Arranging a face-to-face assessment, e.g. home visit, urgent appointment
      with GP, routine appointment with GP, nurse appointment
    Urgent referral to A&E
    Collecting a prescription
    Phoning the patient back later with some further advice
    Organising tests

*Safety net*   Ensure that a robust plan is in place so patient is clear if/when they need to
      contact GP or when you will see them next
    Explain how patient can contact you if they need to, e.g. via telephone or via
      appointment
    Consider referral (e.g. if red flags)

# Home visit

This can be approached as a normal consultation, but with the emphasis shifted to ensuring that the patient is adequately managed at home or referring/arranging for further care as required.

## Data gathering

| | |
|---|---|
| *Preparation* | Familiarise yourself with patient's relevant clinical details prior to visiting |
| | Phone patient prior to visit to ascertain reasons for visit and ICE |
| *Introduce yourself* | "Hello, my name is Dr X. I'm a GP from Y Medical Centre" |
| | "Is there anyone else you want present during my visit?" |
| *Open question(s)* | "How can I help today?" |
| *Targeted history* | As necessary |
| *Social history* | Is patient adequately supported at home? |
| | Is patient able to perform basic activities of daily living? |
| | Does the patient require social services or OT input? |
| *Red flags* | ?Vulnerable patient, ?safeguarding issues |
| *Targeted examination* | As necessary |

## Interpersonal skills

| | |
|---|---|
| *ICE and effect on daily life* | Effect on life and ADLs are especially important |
| | Be sensitive to patient's mood and don't be afraid to ask how they are feeling or if their symptoms are getting them down |
| | ICE early on to understand what is worrying the patient and what they are expecting from you |
| | Allow patient time to ask questions and voice concerns |
| | Summarise / repeat advice |
| | Ask patient to repeat back information to check they have correctly understood |
| | Ensure all patient's concerns have been addressed before ending visit |

# Management

*Investigations*    As appropriate

*Management*    Options include:
Management in primary care
Issuing a prescription – this may need to be delivered to the patient's house
Phoning the patient back later with some further advice
Organising tests
Arranging community support, e.g. specialist/district nursing team, palliative care, CPN
Urgent referral to A&E/secondary care
Ensuring whole patient is being looked at including social needs

*Safety net*    Ensure that a robust follow-up plan is in place and that the patient is clear if/when they when they need to contact GP or when you will see them next
Explain how patient can contact you if they need to, e.g. via telephone or via appointment
Consider referral (e.g. if red flags)

# Breaking bad news

## Data gathering

| | |
|---|---|
| *Preparation* | Ideally should be face-to-face and not via telephone |
| | Ensure quiet, private setting without interruptions |
| | Consider inviting spouse/relative/friend if appropriate |
| | Ensure you are familiar with patient's history and test results |
| *Check patient's understanding* | This is essential for an efficient consultation |
| | *"Before we start, I wanted to ask you...* |
| | *...what is your understanding of the tests and why they were done?"* |
| *Symptoms* | Clarify patient's symptoms if relevant, e.g. diabetes, thyroid |
| | *"How have you been since you were last seen?"* |
| *Warning shot* | This allows the patient to prepare for the bad news |
| | *"Unfortunately the test results have come back ..."* |
| | or |
| | *"Unfortunately the test results do show some abnormal findings"* |
| | *"I'm afraid it looks more serious than we had hoped ..."* |
| | <then pause> |
| *Break news* | *"....they show you have <hyperthyroidism>"* |
| *General health* | PMH, DH, FH |
| *Social history* | Family, relationships |
| | Identify patient's support networks |
| | *"Who's at home?"* Smoking, alcohol |
| | Occupation, driving |
| *Examination* | For example, BP, weight, urine |

## Interpersonal skills

| | |
|---|---|
| *ICE* | Clearly explain diagnosis, avoid jargon, use patient's own words |
| | How much information to give depends on emotional response of patient |
| | Establish the patient's concerns – they are not always what you think they are! |
| *"Chunk 'n' check"* | Give information to patient in smalls "chunks" then "check" their understanding: |
| | *"Do you mind repeating back to me what I've just said to you so that I can check that you have understood?"* |

*"Is this making sense?"*

*"Would you like me to explain more?"*

Don't talk too much, allow patient to gather thoughts and speak

Give time for patient to ask questions

*Empathy*     Acknowledge patient's emotions and feelings

*"It must be difficult for you..."*

Soft caring tone of voice, eye contact, open body language

Offer patient a tissue if tearful

Avoid statements such as *"I know how you feel"* as you cannot know exactly how someone feels. If there is a poor prognosis avoid saying *"There is nothing more we can do"*

It may not be appropriate to go through a more detailed management plan in the context of breaking bad news – use your judgement based on the patient's reaction and understanding

# Management

*Investigations*     As necessary

*Management*     Allow patient to ask questions and express concerns

Negotiate management plan *with* patient

Offer written information

Lifestyle advice, e.g. stop smoking

Conservative, medical, surgical and social management as necessary

*Safety net*     Allow telephone access

Follow up and support is especially important, often multiple consultations required

Suggest bringing along relative/friend/spouse to future consultation or offer to speak to them on the phone

Referral as indicated

[**Note**] Whilst the above is a comprehensive template to use when approaching this case, in real life one of the main issues is that of information overload for the patient. Ensure that you chunk 'n' check and allow time for the patient to process the information in their own way.

As always, ensure you feel comfortable with the wording you use for the 'warning shot' and 'empathy statements' – experiment during practice sessions to find the wording that works for you.

Whilst eye contact can be difficult in these situations, it is an important part of establishing rapport.

A clear follow-up or management plan is essential in helping the patient feel supported.

Practise breaking bad news using jargon-free language. Practising with a non-medic is especially useful for this.

# The angry patient and complaints

*General points*   Actively listen to the complaint
Remain professional and calm
Allow patient to speak and vent their anger

*Acknowledge*   This allows the patient to feel heard and allows them to vent their anger
*and empathise*   Thank the patient: *"Thank you for bringing this to my attention"*
Acknowledge and empathise: *"I can see that it would be very annoying to wait so long"*

*Ask questions*   Be inquisitive and use open questions to find out what has happened. This allows patient to voice their concerns, tell their story and also stops the doctor from being defensive:
*"Could you tell me what's upsetting you?"*

*Concerns*   Find out patient's concerns and address them where possible
Find out specifically if there is anything they want you to do, e.g. *"Is there anything in particular you were hoping I could do?"*

*Apologise*   Even if you have done nothing wrong you can apologise, e.g. *"I'm sorry you had to go through that"*

*Summarise*   Summarise their concern: *"So you waited 10 weeks for the appointment?"*
Summarise the action plan (see below)

*Joint Action*   Emphasise your commitment to helping the patient
*Plan*   Ensure there are no other issues that have not been dealt with
Summarise plan to ensure patient and you agree on actions
- *"I will raise this at a practice meeting"*
- *"Let's see if we can stop this occurring again"*

Direct patient to official complaints procedure if appropriate
- *"Would you like to register a formal complaint?"*

## General approach to case

Take a conciliatory approach
Attempt to de-escalate any conflict
Try not to be defensive or aggressive, e.g. avoid saying *"I have been doing my best. Don't you realise how hard I have been trying?"* which simply escalates the situation
Express empathy, concern and support
Do not blame others, e.g. *"The hospital/nurse is so disorganised"* or *"The receptionist should know better"*

***Body language***   Maintain non-threatening eye contact

Avoid raising your eyebrows, pursing your lips or any aggressive stance.

Consider breaking eye contact from time to time while speaking to
demonstrate your wish to be conciliatory

## Complaints procedure principles in general practice

- The first step is usually for the complainant to write or speak to the practice manager
- Rapid acknowledgement
- Explanation and apology
- How it will be put right
- Complaints procedure in writing on practice leaflet

## The abusive patient

- The patient's need to be heard is balanced against the doctor's right not to be abused or insulted
- "*I am trying to listen to you but can't whilst you are using such bad language*"
- "*Maybe it would be better to do this at another time when you are calmer/being less disruptive*"
- This may need repeating
- An effective phrase in real life is "*Do you realise that you are shouting?*" which can often stop the patient mid-verbal abuse

# Patient refusing emergency management

| | |
|---|---|
| *Capacity* | Does patient have capacity to make *this* decision? E.g. if they are hypoglycaemic or intoxicated they may well not |
| *Give advice* | Clearly explain what your advice is, e.g. *"My advice is to call an ambulance"* |
| *Explain consequences* | Clearly explain consequences of not following advice, e.g. *"You may suffer irreversible heart damage and there is a risk of death"* |
| *Clarify patient's understanding* | This is part of assessing capacity and must be performed for both your advice and consequences – avoid jargon |
| *Repeat* | The advice may need to be repeated |
| *Documentation* | Ensure event fully documented<br>Obtain patient's signature if appropriate |

Tips:
- There is usually no need to adopt a forceful tone of voice, and this often just scares the patient and fuels any denial process.
- Show empathy, use a caring tone of voice, and demonstrate that your advice and efforts are in the patient's best interests.
- Even if the patient refuses admission, try to offer them some form of management, e.g. aspirin or antibiotics.

# Mental Capacity Act

*Came into effect in UK in April 2007*

The Act serves to protect and outline a framework for vulnerable adults who are unable to make decisions for themselves due to lack of mental capacity.

## Mental capacity test

The test for *lacking* mental capacity is in two parts.

To *lack* capacity, patient must:
1. have impairment of mental functioning, *and*
2. be unable to make the decision at the time it needs to be made due to this impairment of mental functioning

To be *able to make a decision*, the person must be able to:
1. <u>understand</u> the information relevant to the decision
2. <u>retain</u> the information relevant to the decision
3. use or <u>weigh</u> the information, or
4. <u>communicate</u> the decision (by any means)

[**Note**] Assessment of mental capacity is specific for each individual decision at a particular time.

## Principles of the Mental Capacity Act

1. A presumption of mental capacity
2. Patient has the freedom to make unwise decisions
3. Patient should be given all appropriate help before they are deemed unable to make decisions on their own behalf
4. If the patient lacks capacity, the decision made on their behalf must:
   - be in the best interests of patient
   - be the least restrictive alternative

[**Note**] If an individual aged 18 or over is deemed not to be competent, nobody else is able to give consent on their behalf. In this scenario clinicians can provide care and treatment in the best interests of the patient.

# Patients under 16

## Competency

Any <u>competent</u> young person, regardless of age, can independently seek medical advice and give valid consent to medical treatment.

At the age of 16 years or over, the person can be presumed to have capacity to consent unless there is evidence to the contrary.

Patients under 16 years old cannot be presumed to be competent to give consent. They can be considered to be competent if they meet the following criteria (this is known as 'Gillick competency'). They must be able to:
- understand the options available – nature, purpose, risks and benefits
- understand the consequences of each treatment, and of non-treatment
- retain and weigh up all the information
- communicate their decision

Competency is decision-specific, i.e. the patient may be competent to make a simple decision but not another more complex one.

If a child is assessed not to be competent, consent would need to be given by a person with parental responsibility (as long as they are also competent).

Even if the patient has competence, best practice is to encourage the patient to speak to parents "...and explore the reasons if the patient is unwilling to do so" (GMC). This also applies to 16 and 17 year olds.

> Explain to the patient that:
> - a doctor is legally obliged to discuss the value of parental support
> - they will respect their confidentiality

[**Note**] A doctor must always act in the best interests of the patient. Emergency treatment can be given to children without consent of child or parents if it prevents death or serious harm to the child.

## Fraser guidelines

These guidelines apply specifically to contraceptive advice for under 16s. Doctors can provide contraceptive advice and treatment without parental consent as long as the following criteria are met:

- the young person understands the doctor's advice
- the young person cannot be persuaded to inform their parents
- the young person is likely to begin, or to continue having, sexual intercourse with or without contraception
- unless the young person receives contraceptive treatment, their physical or mental health, or both, are likely to suffer
- the young person's best interests require them to receive contraceptive advice or treatment with or without parental consent.

[**Note**] Patients have the option of registering with another GP for contraceptive services only.

## Confidentiality

*"The duty of confidentiality owed to a person under 16 is as great as that owed to any other person"*

*BMA, RCGP*

Confidentiality must be respected except in the most exceptional circumstances, for example, where the health, safety or welfare of someone other than the patient would otherwise be at serious risk.

Doctor can breach confidentiality if ALL of below are met:
- the patient does not have sufficient understanding (lacks competence)
- the patient cannot be persuaded to involve an appropriate person in the consultation
- it is in the best interests of the patient

So, even if the patient lacks competence, try to maintain confidentiality unless it is not in the patient's best interests.

In exceptional circumstances where a doctor chooses to break confidentiality, the doctor must:
1. try to convince the patient to voluntarily give information first
2. be prepared to justify his or her decision before the GMC

# Domestic violence

*Based on RCGP guidance*

**Emphasise confidentiality**

**Lead question**    *"Do you ever feel afraid of your partner?"*

**Ask about domestic violence**    *"Have you ever been subject to violence at home?"*

**Allow patient to tell story**

**Establish risk**    Establish risk of harm to patient

Are there any other forms of abuse, e.g. emotional or sexual?

Establish if patient has any children, how old they are, and if they are at risk of being harmed

Are the family already known to social services or are there previous child protection concerns?

**Provide information**    *"Violence in the home is as illegal as violence in the streets"*

**Safety plan**    Do not pressurise into any specific action

Encourage and respect the patient's autonomy

- Accurate documentation is essential.
- Photographs should be taken of all patients with visible injuries.
- It is important to demonstrate care and tact when asking these often very difficult questions.
- Use a warm and caring tone of voice and give the patient time to respond.
- Remain non-judgemental.

# Palliative care

Screen for depression and anxiety (and treat!).

Wellbeing of family/carers – offer support where required, e.g. counselling.

ICE, empathise and pick up on cues.

Remember community palliative care teams, district nurses, Macmillan nurses, local hospices, social services, benefits.

This case may also be a home visit (see **Home Visit** case).

Below is a list of common symptoms. Look for and treat the cause rather than simply prescribing medications where possible. Having said that, treatment options are listed below.

## Pain

*Mild*: paracetamol, ibuprofen.

*Moderate*: Diclofenac 50 mg tds, co-codamol 30/500.

*Severe*: Oramorph = morphine sulphate elixir 10 mg/5 ml
- give with laxative, treat any nausea
- start at 5 mg (2.5 ml) 4-hourly, aim for complete analgesia (no breakthrough pain)
- titrate by increasing dose (not interval)
- once pain control achieved, divide 24 h dose by 2 and give as MST 12-hourly
- as tolerance occurs, add Oramorph (elixir), then total 24 h dose again once control achieved
- use one-sixth of total daily morphine dose for breakthrough pain
- use suppositories, patches or injections if unable to swallow

*Gastric distension*: try antacid or domperidone 10 mg tds.

*Bowel colic*: loperamide or hyoscine hydrobromide.

*Muscle spasm*: baclofen, diazepam.

*Bone pain*: opiates are usually required, NSAIDs, radiotherapy.

*Nerve compression pain*: dexamethasone if due to inflammation, radiotherapy.

*Neuropathic pain*: tricyclic antidepressant, gabapentin, pregabalin.

## Controlled drugs

Know where to look in *BNF*.

# Anorexia

*Causes*: depression, drugs, nausea, obstruction, sore mouth.

*Treatment*: small feeds, small plate, prednisolone 15–30 mg daily.

# Vomiting

*Causes:* obstruction, drugs (chemotherapy, opiates), raised ICP, renal failure, hypercalcaemia.

*Ask about*: headache, micturition, papilloedema, obstruction.

*Investigations*: U&Es, calcium.

*Management*: prochlorperazine (buccal, PO, PR, im), metoclopramide, cyclizine, domperidone.

# Hiccups

Treat any gastric distension with antacid, metoclopramide, baclofen.

Chlorpromazine for intractable hiccups.

# Anxiety

Manage cause, involve carers/district nurse/Macmillan nurses.

Citalopram 20 mg od, diazepam 2–5 mg tds, temazepam for insomnia.

# Constipation

*Causes:* opiates, obstruction, immobility, dehydration.

Beware the patient in overflow, e.g. on morphine with diarrhoea.

*Management:* lactulose, movicol, senna, glycerol suppositories, phosphate enema.

# Cough

*Management:* steam inhalation, codeine linctus, Oramorph.

# Depression

Low index of suspicion, involve carer/district nurse, ensure carers/family well supported.

# Dyspnoea

Exclude pneumonia, effusion, bronchospasm.

Consider prescribing morphine, diazepam.

Secretions: hyoscine, atropine.

Bronchospasm: dexamethasone.

# Hearing impairment

Research shows that this patient group's needs are not often met by healthcare professionals.

For the CSA the case will most likely be a patient who can lip read.

If there is no answer when you call the patient in, stand up and open the door yourself as the patient may not have heard.

| | |
|---|---|
| *Preparation* | Read patient's notes beforehand to avoid looking at notes during consultation |
| *Clarify nature and degree of impairment* | Is the patient completely deaf or is their hearing only moderately impaired? |
| *Clarify preferred method of communication* | Ask how patient would like to be communicated with, e.g. lip reading, sign language (will require interpreter), writing things down |
| *Confirm patient's understanding* | Ask them to repeat what they have understood |
| *For a lip reading patient\** | Face the patient with good lighting on your face so that they can see your lips<br>Speak clearly at normal pace<br>Use whole sentence rather than single word replies because much of lip reading is guess work and relies on context of words within a sentence<br>Do not shout<br>Use gestures, e.g. point or mime where appropriate<br>Provide written information or draw diagrams where possible |

*Based on GMC guidance.

# Learning disability

Learning disability (LD) patients generally have increased health needs but see their GP less often compared with general population (i.e. the 'inverse care law') and often need a multidisciplinary team approach.

## Data gathering

| | |
|---|---|
| *Preparation* | Familiarise yourself with patient's clinical details |
| | Collateral history from individuals who know the patient, e.g. relative, carer, key worker, specialist |
| *Introduce yourself* | |
| *Open question* | |
| *Targeted history* | History may need more focused questions including systems review |
| | Medication review – enquire about side-effects |
| *Social history* | Is patient adequately supported at home? |
| | Is patient able to perform basic activities of daily living? |
| | Does the patient require social services or OT input? |
| *Red flags* | ?Vulnerable patient, ?safeguarding issues |
| *Targeted examination* | |

## Interpersonal skills

| | |
|---|---|
| *ICE and effect on daily life* | Avoid jargon |
| | Effect on life and ADLs are important |
| | Ensure family/carers are also included and supported |
| | Be sensitive to patient's mood and co-existing depression or anxiety |
| | Allow patient time to ask questions and voice concerns |
| | Summarise / repeat advice |
| | Ask patient to repeat back information to check they have correctly understood |

# Management

*Suggested
investigations*

*Management*     Give written information where possible
Health promotion, e.g. lifestyle and dietary advice, smoking cessation
Ensure whole patient is being looked at including social needs
Ensure care between multidisciplinary team is co-ordinated: *"when are
you next going to be seen by specialist?"*
Ensure family / carers are also involved and supported
Book annual health screen with practice nurse if not already done

*Safety net*     Try to ensure follow up with same GP for continuity of care
Explain how patient can contact you if they need to, e.g. via telephone or via
appointment
Consider referral (e.g. if red flags)

# Consultations with more than one person

## Data gathering

| | |
|---|---|
| *Establish who is who* | "So how are you both related to each other?"<br>"How do you know each other?"<br>Avoid leading questions such as *"so are you the patient's mother?"*<br>Ensure you know who the patient is |
| *Establish consent* | Ensure patient is comfortable with third party being present<br>If sensitive information is being discussed, ensure patient gives consent for this to be shared with third party |
| *Establish reasons for attendance* | Ask why third party is present |
| *Targeted history* | |
| *Social history* | |
| *Red flags* | Safeguarding issues, child protection, domestic violence<br>Overbearing/dominating third party |
| *Targeted examination* | Consider asking third party to leave for examination |

## Interpersonal skills

| | |
|---|---|
| *ICE and effect* | Ensure you interact with both people present<br>Involve carers in shared decision-making where appropriate<br>If dominant third party, try to ensure patient's voice is heard<br>Look for cues that patient may be uncomfortable with third party being present, e.g. poor eye contact<br>If you ask third party to leave, ensure that patient is comfortable with this as they may prefer to be accompanied |
| *For patient* | |

# Management

*Suggested investigations*

*Management*   Consider asking to see patient alone for part of consultation if suspecting red flags or any concerns. Emphasise confidentiality. For example, *"Do you mind if I speak to X alone? This is routine for consultations with more than one person/relatives present"*

*Safety net*   Consider arranging follow up with patient alone or with an independent interpreter if third party is acting as interpreter and you have concerns

# Patient who is a healthcare professional

- If the patient is a doctor / GP / nurse / receptionist, the general approach is to treat them more or less as if they were any other patient.
- Avoid jargon where possible, or if you use it be sure to explain what the term means as for any other patient, e.g. *"I know you are a GP, but generally I like to explain everything as if you weren' t a healthcare professional so apologies if I' m describing things too simplistically"*.
- They may be concerned about seeing a specialist who they know, so respect their right to confidentiality and support them in obtaining care from a provider of their choice.
- If they use jargon that you do not understand, do not be afraid to question them because they may have an incomplete understanding themselves of a particular condition.
- In some cases the patient is not obviously a healthcare professional – if you hear a patient using jargon you could ask *"what do you do for a living?"* or *"are you medically trained?"* depending on the situation.

# Section 3
# Typical cases

# Cardiovascular lifestyle advice

*Summary of NICE and Joint British Societies' Guidelines*

|  |  |
|---|---|
| ***Diet*** | • Fat should be <30% of diet <br> • High polyunsaturated fats, low saturated fats <br> • Five portions fruits and vegetables <br> • Do not routinely recommend omega 3, or plant sterols |
| ***Exercise*** | • 30 minutes moderate intensity physical activity a day, at least 5 days a week, or at safe maximum capacity (if co-morbidities), e.g. cycling, brisk walking, stairs. *"Anything that gets your heart rate up"*. <br> • Shorter bouts of physical activity of 10 minutes or more accumulated throughout the day are as effective as longer sessions of activity. <br> • Reduce sedentary behaviour, e.g. watching TV. <br> • Make enjoyable activities daily part of life, e.g. walking to work, or partly walking to work. <br> • Build activity into the day, e.g. using stairs instead of the lift, taking a lunchtime walk. <br> • Agree goals, provide written information. |
| ***Weight loss*** | If BMI >25 |
| ***Smoking cessation*** | See **Smoking cessation** case |
| ***Alcohol*** | 2–3 units/day in women, 3–4 units/day in men <br> Avoid binge drinking |
| ***Avoid salt and caffeine*** | Salt <6g per day |

## Post-MI

- Sexual intercourse when comfortable to do so, usually after 4 weeks; no increase in MI compared to rest of population.
- Encourage cardiac rehabilitation program (stable patients only).
- Driving – not for 1 week post PCI or 4 weeks if no PCI

# Aspirin and prevention of cardiovascular disease

*Based on CKS Guidance (2013)*

### Primary prevention of cardiovascular disease

- That is, if the patient has no prior cardiovascular disease.
- Aspirin is no longer recommended for primary prevention of CVD because the rate of bleeding offsets the cardiovascular prevention benefits.
- Aspirin is not licensed for primary prevention of CVD, including in those patients with diabetes and hypertension.

### Secondary prevention of cardiovascular disease

- That is, if the patient has established cardiovascular disease.
- Daily aspirin is still recommended for secondary prevention of cardiovascular disease for those with angina, and previous MI/CVA/TIA.

### Primary prevention of cardiovascular disease in diabetics

- NHS Clinical Knowledge Summaries states that there is increasing evidence that aspirin is not effective in primary prevention of cardiovascular disease in patients with diabetes.
- SIGN have updated their diabetes guidelines to reflect this, whereas NICE as of yet have not; NICE recommend aspirin in diabetic patients if >50 years or raised CVD risk and BP <145/80. Note that this is an unlicensed use of aspirin which is not licensed for primary prevention of CVD.

# Hypertension

## Data gathering

|  |  |
|---|---|
| *History* | Usually asymptomatic |
|  | *CVD risk factors* |
|  | CVD, DM, smoking, raised cholesterol, family history |
| *Social history* | Smoking, alcohol |
|  | Lifestyle – occupation, stress, diet, exercise |
| *Red flags* | Diastolic BP >120, microscopic haematuria, encephalopathy, pregnant |
|  | Impending complications, e.g. TIA, left ventricular failure |
|  | Papilloedema, retinal haemorrhage |
| *Examination* | Weight |
|  | BP / ABPM / HBPM |
|  | Fundi |
|  | Heart |
|  | Peripheral pulses including aortic aneurysm |

## Interpersonal skills

|  |  |
|---|---|
| *ICE* | Stress, adherence to medications |
| *For patient* | *"What is your understanding of high blood pressure?"* |
|  | *"The top number is the pressure in the arteries when the heart contracts and the lower number is the pressure when the heart is relaxed"* |
|  | *"Do you have any idea why your blood pressure may be high?"* |
|  | *"One of several risk factors that can increase the chance of having a heart attack or stroke"* |
|  | *"There are a variety of factors that can cause high blood pressure such as genetics (or runs in families), stress, lack of exercise and high levels of salt in your diet"* |

## Management

|  |  |
|---|---|
| *Investigations* | Urine: dip for haematuria, send to lab for ACR |
|  | Bloods – U&Es, eGFR, lipids, glucose |
|  | ECG |
|  | Urinary catecholamines if young (phaeochromocytoma) |
|  | Calculate CVD risk, e.g. using QRISK |

**Management**    *Conservative*
        Lifestyle advice, relaxation techniques
        *Medical*
          Age <55 years or non-black: ACE inhibitor is first line
          Age >55 years or black: CCB is first-line, or thiazide diuretic if CCB not tolerated
          Other drugs: ARB, beta blockers, alpha blockers, other diuretics
          Primary prevention – consider statin, e.g. if QRISK >20

**Safety net**    Regular review depending on control and calculate CVD risk
        Refer urgently if suspected malignant hypertension or pregnant
        Refer routinely if young (<40) or multiple risk factors

# NICE Guidelines (2011)

## Definitions

- Stage 1 HTN: BP >140/90 and subsequent ABPM >135/85
- Stage 2 HTN: BP >160/100 and subsequent ABPM >150/95
- Severe HTN: either sBP >180 or dBP >110

## Taking BP reading

- Palpate radial pulse before taking reading. Use manual BP machine if pulse irregularity because automated machines are not accurate in pulse irregularities
- Measure BP in both arms. If >20 mmHg difference between readings on two occasions, use arm with higher reading to measure BP
- Measure BP twice. If readings are not similar, measure for a third time. Take the lowest two readings as clinic BP

## Diagnosing hypertension

- If clinic BP >140/90 then offer ABPM to diagnose HTN
- If patient unable to tolerate ABPM, you can use home monitoring instead
- If BP >180/110 (severe HTN), no need to confirm with ABPM. Consider initiating medication. Ensure no red flags

## Other investigations

These are to look for target organ damage whilst awaiting ABPM results.
- Urine: ACR, dipstick for haematuria
- Bloods: glucose, U&Es, eGFR, lipids
- Fundi (for hypertensive retinopathy)
- ECG – for LVH
- Also calculate CVD risk, e.g. using QRISK tool

## When to treat

Treat stage 1 HTN if <80 years old and one of the following:
- target organ damage
- CVD
- diabetes
- renal disease
- 10 year CVD risk >20%

Treat all with stage 2 HTN

## Medical treatment

- <55 years old – ACE inhibitor is first line
- >55 years old or Afro-Caribbean – CCB is first line with thiazide diuretic if CCB not tolerated
- If thiazide used, use chlortalidone or indapamide in preference to bendroflumethiazide or hydrochlorothiazide (but don't change patients who are already treated with the latter two drugs)

## BP targets

- If <80 years old, BP <140/90 (or ABPM <135/85)
- If >80 years old, BP <150/90 (or ABPM <145/85)

# Hypercholesterolaemia

*Incorporating NICE Guidelines (2008 and 2010)*

## Data gathering

**History**  Data gathering is essentially about quantifying diet and cardiovascular risk
*"Can you tell me about your diet?"*
Identify sources of fat and cholesterol in diet such as full fat dairy and fatty meats
?Fried food
*Past medical history*
Hypertension, CKD, DM, CVD, PVD
*Family history*
CVD with age of onset, raised cholesterol
*Drug history*
Antipsychotics, HIV treatment
*Non-modifiable risk factors*
Male, increasing age, South Asian origin

**Social history**  Smoking, alcohol
Exercise

**Red flags**  Chest pain

**Examination**  Obesity: BMI (or waist circumference or waist:hip ratio)
BP
Tendon xanthomas, xanthelasma

## Interpersonal skills

**ICE**  Important to explore ICE so you can build a shared management plan
*"What's your understanding of what cholesterol/high cholesterol is?"*
How willing is patient to undergo lifestyle modification or take medication?

**For patient**  *"A fatty substance made by liver from the fat eaten in our diet. Everybody needs a small amount of cholesterol."*
*"There is good cholesterol (HDL) and bad cholesterol (LDL)"*
*"Too much can build up in arteries and cause them to narrow."*
*"One of several risk factors that can increase chance of having heart attack or stroke"*
*"Cholesterol can be lowered by improving diet, exercise and medications"*

## Management

*Investigations*    Fasting bloods: lipids, glucose, U&Es, LFTs, TFTs
CK only if muscle symptoms

*Management*    Calculate 10 year CVD risk if primary prevention
*Conservative*
Diet, exercise, smoking cessation (see **Cardiovascular lifestyle advice**)
*Medical*
Statins
Ezetimibe
Fibrates
Also consider aspirin (see **Aspirin and prevention of cardiovascular disease**)
Treat co-morbidities, e.g. hypertension, diabetes
Refer patients with familial hypercholesterolaemia for specialist management

*Safety net*    Measure LFTs at 3 and 12 months after starting statin
Regular review

## Diet

Avoid:
- full fat dairy: butter, lard, ghee, cream, full fat cheeses
- fatty meats, e.g. meat pies, sausages

Less frying and roasting: try steaming, grilling, boiling instead.

## Medical treatment

Primary prevention: give statins (NICE: simvastatin 40 mg is first line) for high risk individuals, i.e.:
- 10 year CVD risk >20%
- diabetic
- familial hypercholesterolaemia
- >75 years old – assume these patients are at high CVD risk and consider statin treatment
- lower threshold for initiating statin if (NICE Guidelines):
  - age >75 years
  - South Asian
  - first degree relative with premature CHD
  - rheumatoid arthritis, SLE, CKD, HIV treatment, antipsychotics

Secondary prevention: give statins (NICE: simvastatin 40 mg is first line) for those with established cardiovascular disease (MI, angina, TIA, stroke, PVD):
- aim for total cholesterol <4.0 and LDL cholesterol <2.0 for secondary prevention only (NICE)
- consider increasing to simvastatin 80 mg if not achieved with simvastatin 40 mg (NICE)
- consider atorvastatin if target still not achieved

# Chest pain

*Based on NICE Guidelines (2010)*

## Data gathering

**History**   Pain history, rest pain, trauma
*Symptoms*
SOB, pallor, cough, rash, vomiting, abdominal pain
Leg/calf pain, haemoptysis
*Risk factors*
Smoking, COCP, recent surgery/flight/immobility, past medical history/
family history
*Previous investigations of chest pain*

**Social history**   Smoking, alcohol, recreational drugs

**Red flags**   ACS:
- new onset "cardiac pain"
- "cardiac pain" lasting longer than 15 minutes if known angina
- unstable angina

Haemodynamic instability
Pulmonary oedema
PE
Aneurysm

**Examination**   BP, pulse, temperature, respiratory distress
Heart, lungs, abdomen
Chest wall tenderness, rash
Legs: DVT, oedema

## Interpersonal skills

**ICE**   Effect on life

## Management

**Investigations**   Bloods: FBC, U&Es, LFTs, ESR/CRP, glucose, cardiac enzymes
ECG
CXR

**Management**   Treat as per cause
Don't forget musculo-skeletal and gastro-intestinal causes (e.g. GORD)

*Safety net*    Refer urgently to A&E (by ambulance) if red flags
                    NICE recommends same day referral if no current chest pain but suspected
                      ACS symptoms within last 72 hours
                    If cardiac sounding chest pain stopped >72 hours ago, consider Rapid
                      Access Chest Pain Clinic referral
                    If pain not improving or worsening to seek medical attention

## Case notes

The following symptoms may indicate an ACS:
- chest pain lasting more than 15 minutes
- chest pain associated with nausea and vomiting, marked sweating or SOB
- chest pain with haemodynamic instability
- new onset chest pain
- an abrupt deterioration in stable angina, with frequently recurring pain on minimal exertion

Immediate medical management of suspected ACS in general practice:
- GTN spray
- aspirin 300 mg

Investigations of suspected ACS in general practice (if available)
- ECG (give copy to ambulance/A&E, normal ECG does <u>not</u> exclude ACS).
- Monitor pulse oximetry and heart rhythm.
- Give oxygen if sats <94% on air (if patient has COPD, maintain sats at 88–92% to prevent risk of hypercapnic respiratory failure).

# Angina

*Based on NICE Guidelines (2012)*

## Data gathering

| | |
|---|---|
| *History* | Relief with GTN |
| | Frequency, previous episodes |
| | *Past medical history* |
| | Hypertension, hypercholesterolaemia, DM |
| | *Family history* |
| | Cardiovascular disorders, smoking |
| *Social history* | Smoking, alcohol |
| | Stress |
| *Red flags* | Pain lasting >15 minutes |
| | Unstable angina: rest pain, increasing frequency attacks, pain on minimal exertion |
| | Suspected MI |
| | Haemodynamic instability |
| | Pulmonary oedema |
| *Examination* | BP, pulse |
| | Weight |
| | Heart, ankles |

## Interpersonal skills

| | |
|---|---|
| *ICE* | Effect on life, occupation |
| *For patient* | *"Pain that comes from the heart due to narrowing of its blood vessels. This reduces the blood supply to the heart"* |
| | *"The blood supply may be sufficient to supply the heart muscle at rest, but it may not be enough during exertion"* |

## Management

| | |
|---|---|
| *Investigations* | Bloods – FBC, U&Es, TFTs, cholesterol, glucose |
| | ECG, exercise ECG |
| | CXR |

**Management**    *Conservative*
Stop smoking
Diet, exercise, stress reduction
Inform DVLA (unable to hold HGV licence)
*Medical*
Symptom relief:
- GTN spray for immediate relief (or prior to activities that precipitate symptoms)
- first-line = beta blocker or CCB
- second-line = beta blocker and CCB
- third-line if above not working, e.g. long-acting nitrate, then refer to cardiology

Prevention of new vascular events (secondary prevention):
- aspirin
- statin
- BP control

*Revascularisation*
- Coronary artery bypass graft
- Percutaneous intervention

**Safety net**    Inform patient to seek medical attention immediately if red flags
If unstable angina give GTN spray and aspirin 300 mg and refer as emergency to hospital
Refer if considering revascularisation or not responding to medical treatment
Refer newly diagnosed to Rapid Access Chest Pain Clinic to confirm diagnosis

# Case notes

### Typical angina is (NICE 2010):
- a constricting pain in the front of the chest, neck, jaw or arms
- brought on by exertion
- relieved by rest or GTN in approximately 5 minutes
- may also be brought on by emotion

### Stable angina is unlikely if the pain is (NICE 2010):
- continuous or prolonged
- unrelated to activity
- worse on inspiration
- associated with palpitations, dizziness, tingling or odynophagia

### Using GTN spray (NICE 2012):
- Be able to demonstrate how to use it
- Repeat dose after 5 minutes if pain is not gone
- Call emergency ambulance if pain not gone 5 minutes after second dose

# Palpitations

## Data gathering

**History**  *"What do you mean by palpitations?"*
*"Are you experiencing palpitations now?"*
When does it happen? How long last for?
How fast? Regular/irregular? Ask patient to tap out rhythm
*Associated symptoms*
Cardiovascular: chest pain, SOB, sweating, loss of consciousness/feeling faint
Anxiety: finger and peri-oral tingling (hyperventilation), clarify anxiety symptoms
Fever, pregnancy, menopause
*Past medical history/family history*
Cardiovascular risk factors, anxiety
*Drug history*
Salbutamol, nasal decongestants, thyroxine
Including withdrawal (e.g. benzodiazepine withdrawal)

**Social history**  Caffeine, alcohol, smoking (especially cigars), recreational drugs (e.g. amphetamine)
Stress, anxiety
Occupation
Driving

**Red flags**  Chest pain/MI, syncope, known cardiovascular disease
Family history of sudden death (cardiomyopathy)

**Examination**  BP, pulse
Anaemia
Radio-radial delay, cardiovascular examination
Signs of heart failure
Signs of thyroid disease

## Interpersonal skills

**ICE**  Explore patient's ideas and concerns, effect on life
Anxiety – could be cause or effect

**For patient**  *"Awareness of your own heart beating"*

# Management

*Investigation*   Bloods: FBC, TFTs, glucose, cholesterol
ECG, 24 hour ECG
Echo if suspect cardiomyopathy

*Management*   Treat as per cause
Avoid triggers
Treat any anxiety
Reassure if simple occasional ectopic beats and no evidence of CHD with normal investigations
Notify DVLA if syncope or cardiac cause

*Safety net*   Refer as per cause
Urgent referral if:
- suspect VT
- current palpitations with SOB / chest pain / syncope / hypotension

# Intermittent claudication

*Based on NICE Guidelines (2012)*

## Data gathering

| | |
|---|---|
| *History* | Cramping pain in buttock/thigh/calf on walking, relieved by rest |
| | Claudication distance |
| | *Cardiovascular risk factors* |
| | CVD, DM, raised cholesterol, family history |
| *Social history* | Smoking |
| *Red flags* | Critical ischaemia: rest pain, pallor, paraesthesiae, gangrene |
| *Examination* | BP, pulse, weight |
| | Heart |
| | Legs: temperature, skin, infections/ulcers |
| | Know how to examine peripheral pulses |
| | Ankle brachial pressure index |

## Interpersonal skills

| | |
|---|---|
| *ICE* | Effect on life |
| *For patient* | *"Pain due to narrowing in arteries that supply blood to legs"* |

## Management

| | |
|---|---|
| *Investigations* | Bloods: FBC, U&Es, cholesterol, glucose |
| | ECG |
| | Ankle brachial pressure index or Doppler studies |
| *Management* | *Conservative* |
| | Smoking cessation |
| | Supervised exercise programme |
| | Diet |
| | Foot care – podiatry, regular self-inspection |
| | *Medical* |
| | Cardiovascular prevention – aspirin or clopidogrel, statin, BP |
| | *Surgical* |
| | If red flags or treatment resistant |
| | Options include stenting, angiography and bypass graft |
| *Safety net* | Refer if red flags or interfering with functioning |

**Remember: risk to the limb is low, risk to life is high** (i.e. people die from MIs and CVAs; primary prevention is the main treatment)

# Varicose veins

*Based on NICE Guidelines (2013)*

## Data gathering

| | |
|---|---|
| *History* | Pain, aching, itching |
| | Cosmetic appearance and effect on life |
| | Is patient planning to have more children? |
| | *Risk factors* |
| |    Prolonged standing, obesity, pregnancy |
| | *Past medical history* |
| |    Ulceration or phlebitis, DVT |
| | *Drug history* |
| |    COCP, HRT |
| *Social history* | Occupation – may involve prolonged standing |
| | Smoking, alcohol |
| *Red flags* | DVT, abdominal mass |
| *Examination* | BMI |
| | Abdomen |
| | Varicose veins: long vs. short saphenous distribution, thrombophlebitis |
| | Venous insufficiency: varicose eczema, ulceration, haemosiderin deposition |
| | Superficial venous thrombosis (hard painful veins) |

## Interpersonal skills

| | |
|---|---|
| *ICE* | *"Why have you come to see a doctor now?"* |
| | Explore patient's concerns and expectations |
| | Possible effect on self esteem |
| *For patient* | *"Enlarged or dilated superficial veins"* |
| | *"Common, affects up to one-third of the population"* |
| | *"Usually do not cause any problems or complications from a medical point of view"* |

## Management

| | |
|---|---|
| *Investigations* | Ultrasound studies |
| *Management* | *Conservative* |
| | Reassurance that most do not cause problems |
| | Weight loss, walking/exercise, avoid prolonged standing, elevate legs when possible |
| | Support stockings |

*Surgical*

Refer to vascular surgeons if:

- symptomatic
- signs of venous insufficiency or venous ulceration / Hx of venous ulceration
- superficial venous thrombosis

Surgical options include, e.g. injection, avulsion, stripping, laser therapy

Surgical treatment not given on NHS for purely cosmetic reasons – refer to local criteria

## Safety net

[**Note**] Surgery is usually reserved for women who have no further plans to have children to prevent recurrence during pregnancy.

# Smoking cessation

## Data gathering

*History*  "*How much do you smoke?*"
"*What do you smoke?*" (e.g. cigarettes, pipe, roll-ups)
When does the patient smoke? e.g. work, social
When did they start smoking? Why?
Have they quit previously? Why did they restart?
*Past medical history/family history*
　　DM, hypertension, hypercholesterolaemia, obesity, cancer
*Drug history*
　　Contraindications to treatment: epilepsy, psychiatric history

*Social history*  Any smokers at home/work/in relationship?
Stress at home/work/in relationship?
Support groups

*Previous attempts*  What happened?
What tried?
Any problems with previous treatment?

*Motivation*  "*Why do you want to give up?*"
"*Why now?*"
"*Has anything happened to make you want to give up?*"
"*Have you got a particular quit date in mind?*"

## Interpersonal skills

*ICE*  "*Was there anything in particular you were hoping I could do?*" e.g. patient
may want alternative therapies or hypnotherapy
Does the patient have support and motivation in his relationships to help
him quit?

## Management

*Management*  "*Do you know what treatment options are available?*"
Encourage patient to agree on a stop date
*Conservative*
　　Self-help, encouragement, support groups
　　Local stop-smoking service

*Medical*
> NRT: patches, gum, inhalers, nasal spray
> Bupropion (Zyban)
> Varenicline (Champix)
> *"All medical treatments are more effective in combination with behavioural treatment"*

**Safety net**    Regular follow up and support

## Bupropion (Zyban)

8 week course
Side-effects: dry mouth, insomnia
Contraindicated in patients:
- with history of seizures or eating disorders
- experiencing symptoms of acute alcohol or benzodiazepine withdrawal

## Varenicline (Champix)

12 week course
Side-effects: nausea, insomnia, abnormal dreams
Should not be used if under 18, pregnant or breastfeeding
Can cause mood changes and suicidal ideation, so use with caution in psychiatric conditions
NICE Guidance (2007) states varenicline should only be prescribed:
- as part of programme with behavioural support
- and if smoker has expressed desire to quit

## E-cigarettes

- These are electrical devices that mimic cigarette smoking and often contain nicotine
- They may be safer than normal cigarettes
- We do not know long-term effects of the vapour on body and they are not proven as being safe
- They are not regulated so you cannot be sure what you are inhaling
- No proof that they can help stop smoking

# Cough

*Based on CKS Guidelines (2012)*

## Data gathering

*History*  Sputum and colour, frequency, diurnal variation
*Associated symptoms*
SOB, wheeze, chest pain, fever, nasal congestion
GI symptoms (GORD)
Leg oedema or pain (CCF/PE)
*Environment*
Precipitant, exercise tolerance, allergy, pets, dust
Travel, contacts, stress
*Past medical history/family history*
PE/DVT, GORD, atopy (hayfever, asthma, eczema)
*Drug history*
ACE inhibitor

*Social history*  Smoking
Occupation
Stress – can patient cope at home?

*Red flags*  Lung cancer: haemoptysis, weight loss, >3 weeks of chest/shoulder pain, SOB, hoarseness, clubbing, cervical/supraclavicular lymphadenopathy
TB: weight loss, fever, night sweats, anorexia, clubbing.

*Examination*  BP, weight
PEFR
Pulse, respiratory rate, clubbing, anaemia/cyanosis
Sinus tenderness, throat, neck/lymph nodes, chest, heart
Legs if suspect PE/CCF

## Interpersonal skills

*ICE*  Effect on sleep, exercise, job
Sensitively inform patient if you suspect this could be cancer; this can be done by exploring patient's concerns and demonstrating empathy

## Management

*Investigations*  Bloods: FBC, U&Es, LFTs, ESR/CRP
Sputum MCS

ECG: CCF, PE
Spirometry
CXR, CT chest

*Management*   Treat cause
Smoking cessation

*Safety net*   If ?lung cancer refer under 2 week rule and arrange CXR
If ?TB arrange CXR, 3 sputum samples for AFBs and culture, refer TB clinic
within 2 weeks

# Causes of cough

| Chronic cough (>4 weeks) | Acute cough |
|---|---|
| Asthma (nocturnal often)<br>Cancer of the bronchus<br>Gastro-oesophageal reflux<br>COPD<br>TB<br>Post-nasal drip<br>ACE inhibitors | URTI<br>LRTI/pneumonia<br>PE<br>CCF<br>Asthma |

*URTI (based on CKS & NICE Guidelines):*
- Rest and oral fluids
- Paracetamol or ibuprofen prn for pain or malaise
- Smoking cessation
- Antibiotics are not likely to be helpful and may cause side-effects such as diarrhoea, vomiting or a rash
- Cough medicines may help but no more effective than honey and lemon drink
- Tell patient that the average duration of a cough is 3 weeks and to see GP if cough persists longer than this. Note that average duration of common cold is 1.5 weeks.

# COPD

*Based on NICE Guidelines (2010)*

## Data gathering

**History**  Consider COPD if persistent:
- cough >1 month
- sputum: colour and volume
- SOB: ?exertional

*Exacerbations*
How many, time course, symptoms, severity
Recent admissions

*Co-morbidities*
Depression screen, anxiety screen
Generally fit and well? Appetite? Exercise tolerance?
Waking at night* (may suggest asthma)

**Social history**  Smoking, passive smoking
Occupational*: exposure to dusts/chemicals

**Red flags**  Non-smoker with family history
Weight loss, haemoptysis, focal chest signs including chest pain
<40 years old
Severe SOB

**Examination**  BMI – weight, height
Clubbing, anaemia, right ventricular failure/cor pulmonale, ankle swelling, lungs
FEV1 and FVC
Inhaler technique
MRC Dyspnoea score
Oxygen sats

## Interpersonal skills

**ICE**  *"How does this affect your daily life?"*
*"Does it stop you doing anything in particular?"*
*"Does it limit your ability to exercise?"*
*"Is there any reason you have come to see me now?"*
*"How are you coping at home?"*
*"How well are the inhalers working?"*

*"Do you know which inhalers to use when?"*
Non-judgemental if patient smokes

**For patient**  *"Airflow into lungs is obstructed. This is due to lung damage, usually caused
    by smoking"*
*"Stopping smoking is the most important and effective treatment"*
*"Inhalers can be used to ease symptoms and treat flare-ups"*
*"Could I please see how you use your inhalers?"*
*"Could you talk me through when you use each inhaler?"*

# Management

**Investigations**  Bloods: FBC* (anaemia or polycythaemia), U&Es, ESR, LFTs, cholesterol,
    glucose
Refer for post-bronchodilator spirometry for diagnosis
CXR* (for anyone with chronic cough to exclude lung cancer/other
    pathology)

**Management**  *Conservative*
    Smoking cessation = "*the most effective treatment*"
    Weight loss, exercise
    Pulmonary rehabilitation/chest physiotherapy
*Medical*
    Short-acting bronchodilators
    Long-acting bronchodilators
    Inhaled corticosteroids (ensure never given as monotherapy)
    Theophylline
    Mucolytics
*Other*
    Vaccinations: influenza, pneumococcal
    LTOT
    Surgery

**Safety net**  Regular review
Think about palliative care needs
Refer to chest physician if:
• <40 years old
• non-smoker
• severe SOB
• diagnostic uncertainty
• haemoptysis, cor pulmonale, considering LTOT or surgery

*As per NICE Guidelines (2010)

# Summary of NICE Guidelines (2010) on COPD

Consider COPD in any smoker >35 years with any of:

- chronic cough
- regular sputum
- exertional SOB
- wheeze
- frequent winter "bronchitis"

The following features suggest asthma rather than COPD:

- chronic unproductive cough
- diurnal or day-to-day variation of breathlessness
- waking at night due to SOB/wheeze

Diagnosis is with post-bronchodilator spirometry:

- diagnose COPD with FEV1:FVC <70%
- FEV1 % predicted gives guide to disease severity
- reversibility (>400 ml after 200 µg salbutamol) suggests asthma
- record both percentages and absolute values

## General management

- Offer pulmonary rehabilitation to all (and those who have been recently admitted with an exacerbation).
- Lifestyle: smoking cessation, treat obesity or low weight, exercise.
- Depression screen.
- Vaccinations: influenza, pneumococcal.

## Stepwise management

In general only continue medical treatments if there is an improvement after 4 weeks as none improve disease survival (i.e. only give symptomatic relief +/− reduce hospital admissions).

1. Short-acting bronchodilator prn (e.g. salbutamol or ipratropium). Salbutamol has the advantage that it can be continued at all steps prn.
2. *Long-acting antimuscarinic (e.g. tiotropium) – don't forget to stop any short-acting antimuscarinic.
3. Long-acting antimuscarinic AND long-acting beta-2 agonist AND inhaled corticosteroid
4. Theophylline or referral.

*Alternatives at this step are:

a. If mild–moderate disesase (i.e. FEV1 >50% predicted) can use long-acting beta-2 agonist (e.g. salmeterol). If this is not enough then proceed to long-acting beta-2 and inhaled steroid combination inhaler.

b. If severe–very severe disease (i.e. FEV1 <50% predicted) can use long-acting beta-2 and inhaled steroid combination inhaler OR can use long-acting beta-2 and long-acting antimuscarinic together if inhaled steroid not tolerated.

### Delivery method

Ensure good inhaler technique.

Spacers should not be cleaned more than once a month (water, washing up liquid and air dry).

Nebulisers if severe or distressing SOB despite maximum inhaler therapy; allow patient to choose face mask. Continue nebulisers only if there is improvement in symptoms.

Trial of inhaled steroids for 4 weeks:
- if FEV1 <50% predicted and >2 exacerbations/year (and symptoms not controlled with bronchodilators)
- continue only if benefit after 4 weeks
- NICE advises to be aware of risk of non-fatal pneumonia in those receiving inhaled steroids
- inhaled steroids should always be used in combination with other drugs, especially long-acting beta-2 agonists

Mucolytics (carbocysteine) if chronic cough/sputum:
- continue only if benefit after 4 weeks
- caution in peptic ulceration – may disrupt stomach lining

### Treatment of exacerbation

- Increase bronchodilators.
- If purulent sputum give antibiotics, e.g. amoxicillin 1 week then co-amoxiclav, macrolide or ciprofloxacin 2nd line for 1 week if no improvement.
- If symptoms affect ADLs give prednisolone 30 mg for 5 days.

Admit to hospital if unwell (e.g. confused, cyanosed, very short of breath), no improvement on treatment, unable to cope at home, already on LTOT, sats <90%.

### Encourage self-management

Give supply of oral steroids and antibiotics to keep at home. Use:
- oral steroids if increased SOB interferes with ADLs.
- antibiotics if purulent sputum.

### Consider referring for LTOT assessment if any of following:

- oxygen sats <92%
- very severe disease (especially if FEV1 <30% predicted)
- cyanosis
- polycythaemia
- peripheral oedema
- raised JVP

LTOT:
- home oxygen 15 h/day (improves survival)

- if used inappropriately can cause respiratory depression in COPD
- warn about fire and explosion risk if they smoke
- can be ambulatory
- if hypercapneic or acidotic on LTOT, consider NIV

Short-burst oxygen therapy:
- can be used for episodes of severe breathlessness if otherwise unresponsive

### Surgery
- Bullectomy, lung volume reduction surgery, lung transplant.

### Cor pulmonale
- Investigate with ECG and echo.
- May need LTOT.
- Diuretic for oedema.
- Not recommended: ACEi, CCBs, alpha-blockers.

# Asthma

*Based on the SIGN/British Thoracic Society Guidelines (2012)*

## Data gathering

|  |  |
|---|---|
| *History* | Nocturnal cough, wheeze, SOB, chest tightness |
|  | Exercise tolerance |
|  | Triggers/allergens |
|  | *Past medical history* |
|  |    Exacerbations, hospital admissions, ITU admissions |
|  | *Family history* |
|  |    Atopy: asthma, eczema, hayfever |
|  | *Drug history* |
|  |    Current medications and how often used |
|  |    Use of spacer |
|  |    Compliance |
|  |    Aspirin, NSAIDs, beta blockers |
| *Social history* | Smoking – active and passive |
|  | Occupation |
|  | *Allergens*: pets, diet |
| *Red flags* | Respiratory distress, silent chest, chest pain, uncontrolled symptoms |
| *Examination* | BMI – weight, height |
|  | PEFR |
|  | Chest |
|  | Cushingoid appearance |
|  | Inhaler/spacer technique |

## Interpersonal skills

|  |  |
|---|---|
| *ICE* | Effect on life: sleep, work, school, sport |
| *For patient* | *"From time to time the airways narrow making it difficult to breathe. This is due to airway inflammation of unknown cause, but medications can prevent this happening"* |
|  | *"Could I please see how you use your inhalers?"* |
|  | *"Could you talk me through when you use each inhaler?"* |

# Management

*Investigations*   PEFR diary (15% variability over 2 weeks)
Spirometry: FEV1:FVC should be <70% in asthma
Trial of bronchodilator/steroid (15% improvement in PEFR)

*Management*   *Conservative*
Smoking cessation, weight loss, allergen avoidance
Education, e.g. "preventers vs. relievers"
Compliance
Inhaler technique – offer training if appropriate
*"If we could make one thing better for your asthma, what would it be?"*
*Medical (adults)*
Step 1: short-acting beta-2 agonist as required
Step 2: ICS
Step 3: long-acting beta-2 agonist
Step 4: high dose ICS or 4th drug, e.g. leukotriene receptor antagonist
Step 5: oral corticosteroid
Short-acting beta-2 agonists immediately prior to exercise if exercise-induced

*Safety net*   Admit to hospital if any respiratory distress
Regular follow up
Refer if uncontrolled symptoms or suspicion of occupational asthma

# Summary of SIGN/British Thoracic Society Guidelines (2012) on Asthma

## Diagnosis

- Diagnosis is clinical – reversible symptoms without alternative explanation.
- No need for investigations if high probability based on clinical assessment.
- For children <5 years of age: difficult to diagnose – try watchful waiting or trial therapy.

### Clinical features raising probability of asthma

- Symptoms worse:
  - at night and early morning
  - after exercise, allergen exposure, cold air
  - after aspirin or beta blockers
- History or family history of atopy.

### Not typical of asthma

- No response to trial asthma therapy.
- Normal examination/PEFR when symptomatic.

- Symptoms with URTI only, with no interval symptoms (e.g. viral-induced wheeze in children).
- Isolated/chronic cough with no wheeze or SOB.
- Change in voice.
- Significant smoking history.

# Prevention

- Breastfeeding *may* have protective effect on child, and so should be encouraged due to other beneficial effects.
- Passive smoking increases risk of wheezing in infancy and asthma.

# Treatment

### Medical stepwise treatment (adults)

Step 1: short-acting beta-2 agonist as required.
Step 2: add ICS.
Step 3: add long-acting beta-2 agonist.
Step 4: add high dose ICS or 4th drug, e.g. leukotriene receptor antagonist.
Step 5: add oral corticosteroid.
Step 6: refer for specialist care.

### Exertional symptoms

Are usually symptomatic of poor control:
- ensure an appropriate treatment including inhaled corticosteroids
- short-acting beta-2 agonists immediately prior to exercise

### Exacerbations managed in community (adults)

- Salbutamol prn +/– spacer.
- Add Prednisolone 40–50 mg daily for at least 5 days.
- Routine antibiotic prescription not indicated.
- For pregnant and breastfeeding women, do not withhold steroids if required and treat as normal.

### Delivery devices

- Patients require training in use of delivery devices upon new prescription.
- Inhaler with spacer for mild exacerbations in adults or children.
- Inhaler with spacer often good for children under 12, especially children under 5.
- Patient preference should be taken into account.

### Little evidence for treatment of asthma with the following

- Nutritional supplements, certain baby formulas or probiotics/microbial exposure.
- Homeopathy, Chinese medicines, acupuncture.
- Air ionisers.

# Obesity

*Based on NICE Guidelines (2006) and SIGN Guidelines (2010)*

## Data gathering

| | |
|---|---|
| *History* | *"Why do you want to lose weight?"* <br> Previous attempts? |
| *CVD risk factors* | HTN, high cholesterol, DM, family history of CVD |
| *Social history* | Smoking, job, exercise, diet |
| *Red flags* | Eating disorder, e.g. binge-eating <br> BMI >40 – very significant effect on life expectancy |
| *Examination* | BP, BMI, waist (at level of anterior superior iliac spine) |

## Interpersonal skills

| | |
|---|---|
| *ICE* | Depression, low self-esteem, stress <br> Binge eating |
| *For patient* | *"What do you think of your size/weight?"* <br> *"Would you like help in losing weight?"* <br> *"Is there any particular reason why you would like to lose weight (now)?"* <br> e.g. perhaps a friend or relative said something ... |

## Management

| | |
|---|---|
| *Investigations* | Urine – glucose <br> Bloods – U&E, LFT, glucose, cholesterol, TSH, LH/FSH |
| *Management* | *"Energy you use must be more than energy you eat"* <br> *Conservative* <br>     Support and encouragement <br>     Diet/dietician <br>     Exercise <br>     Weight management programmes <br> *Medical* <br>     Drugs – orlistat <br> *Surgical* <br>     Bariatric surgery |
| *Follow up* | Weigh no more than weekly, regular follow up |

# Summary of SIGN Guidelines (2010) on obesity

## BMI (weight/height², kg/m²)

18.5–25 =  normal
>25     =  overweight
>30     =  obese (grade 1 obesity = 30–34; grade 2 obesity = 35–40)
>40     =  morbidly obese (= grade 3 obesity)

## For South Asian, Chinese and Japanese patients (SIGN and WHO)

18–23   =  normal
>23     =  overweight
>27.5   =  obese

## Obese patients are at increased risk of:

- cardiovascular risk factors: hypertension, raised cholesterol
- cardiovascular disease
- type 2 diabetes
- arthritis
- varicose veins
- worsening of asthma/COPD symptoms

## Support

- "*10% weight loss will give significant health improvements*" = motivation.
- Improves self-esteem and sense of wellbeing.
- Take slowly and set realistic long-term goals.
- Encourage regular self-weighing.

## Weight-management programmes

- May include psychological/behavioural component.
- These should also be available to people with binge-eating disorders.

## Diet

- Encourage wholegrains, cereals, fruits, vegetables and salads.
- Five portions of fruit and vegetables per day.
- Grilled + boiled + baked rather than fried.
- Smaller portions, limit snacks.
- Less alcohol.
- Water instead of sugary drinks.

## Exercise

- 30 minutes per day for 5 days each week for normal healthy person. This may need to be increased to 45–60 minutes in overweight or obese people.
- Walking, cycling, group activities such as aerobics.
- "Exercise prescription" – for local health services.

- Reduce sedentary behaviour, e.g. watching TV.
- Making enjoyable activities a daily part of life, e.g. walking to work, or partly walking to work.
- Building activity into the day, e.g. using stairs instead of the lift, taking a lunchtime walk.
- Ensure activity is safe and appropriate with gradual increases in activity levels.

### Children

- BMI centile charts are used for children.
- Obesity = BMI >98th centile.
- Weight maintenance is the usual treatment goal.
- Refer if serious co-morbidities or suspicion of endocrine/underlying abnormality (often child has associated short stature).
- Full fat foods should be used up to at least age of 2 years.
- From age 5 onwards and adults, use the eatwell plate (www.eatwell.gov.uk).

# Drugs and surgery for obesity

## Anti-obesity drugs

Use in conjunction with lifestyle measures, set target 5% weight loss over 3 months.

### Orlistat (Xenical) – better for those with high fat intake

- *"Lowers fat absorption"*.
- TDS with or before meals.
- NICE criteria: BMI >30 or >28 with co-morbidity (Type-2 DM, cholesterolaemia, hypertension).
- Continue >12 weeks only if 5% weight loss.
- Can cause reduced absorption of fat-soluble vitamins (A, D, E, K) and reduced COCP efficacy.

*CI*: malabsorption, breastfeeding.
*SEs*: flatulence, diarrhoea.

### Sibutramine (Reductil)

This has been withdrawn from the market after it was found to increase cardiovascular events and stroke.

### Rimonabant (Acomplia)

This has been withdrawn from the market after concerns regarding increased suicidal ideation, depression and other side-effects.

## Bariatric surgery

- NICE criteria: only if BMI >40 or >35 with co-morbidities and other measures failed.
- SIGN criteria: should have completed a structured weight management programme with weight improvement first.
- Needs long-term commitment and follow up.
- Only works alongside conservative and medical measures.
- Monitoring and post-operative follow up required, including:
  - routine bloods: FBC, LFTs, calcium, magnesium, phosphate
  - may need multivitamin, iron and calcium supplements

# Dyspepsia

## Data gathering

**Pain**  Relationship to eating/lying down
Night symptoms, sleep disturbance
*Associated symptoms*
    Vomiting/nausea, bloating, burping, chronic cough, taste in mouth

**History**  *Past medical history*
    Previous endoscopy/investigations
    *H. pylori* infection
*Family history*
    Ulcer, cancer, surgery
*Drug history*
    NSAIDs, SSRIs, steroids, nitrates, Ca antagonists, bisphosphonates
*Social history*
    Lifestyle: alcohol, smoking, appetite, diet, exercise

**Red flags**  >55 years, weight loss, bleeding (PO/PR/melaena), anaemia symptoms
Dysphagia, vomiting, abdominal mass

**Examination**  Weight/BMI
Hands, anaemia, abdomen

## Interpersonal skills

**ICE**  Effect on sleep, work
Asking about lifestyle factors such as diet, stress, smoking and alcohol are
    often key to eliciting the cause
*"Do you have any idea what could be causing the symptoms?"*

## Management

**Investigations**  FBC, LFT, CRP, coeliac screen – consider before referral
Test and treat for *Helicobacter pylori*
Upper GI endoscopy, e.g. if red flags

**Management**  *Conservative*
    Stress, diet, weight reduction
    Smoking, alcohol, caffeine reduction
    Stop NSAIDs, etc.

*Medical*
> Gaviscon / Peptac / Gastrocote
> Proton pump inhibitor for 1–2 months
> Can add $H_2$ antagonist or domperidone
> Consider *H. pylori* test and treat

***Safety net***    Referral if red flags or persistent symptoms
> Consider alternative diagnoses, e.g. gallstones
> Review in 6 weeks if symptoms not improving, or before if symptoms
>> worsening despite treatment

# *H. pylori*

- Can initially test serology or faecal antigen (both require 2 weeks without PPI and 4 weeks without antibiotics for greater test accuracy). Note that serology can remain positive even after eradication for over 12 months.
- Urea breath test to confirm eradication (can prescribe on FP10).
- Treatment – triple therapy with PPI and 2 antibiotics, e.g. lansoprazole 30 mg + amoxicillin 1 g bd + clarithromycin 500 mg bd for 7 days.

## GORD

- Worse lying flat, acid taste in mouth, can cause chronic cough/nocturnal cough.
- Elevate head of bed, avoid late eating, smaller meals (medical treatment as above).
- Diet – avoid fatty foods, alcohol, coffee, citrus fruits.

## Upper GI endoscopy

- *"A thin flexible tube is passed down your food pipe to view your stomach"*.
- No PPIs or $H_2$ receptor blockers for at least 2 weeks beforehand.

# Irritable bowel syndrome

*Based on NICE Guidelines (2008)*

Very common – 10–20% prevalence.

Emphasis on positive diagnosis rather than exclusion of disease.

## Data gathering

*Symptoms*     Consider IBS if 6 months of:
>    <u>A</u>bdominal pain
>    <u>B</u>loating
>    <u>C</u>hange in bowel habit

IBS must have either (positive diagnosis):
>    1.  relief of pain with defecation
>    2.  altered stool frequency/form (straining, urgency, incomplete evacuation)

Also: symptoms worse after eating, PR mucus

*Red flags*     Weight loss, bleeding, nocturnal symptoms, masses (rectal/abdominal)
Change in bowel habit for 6 weeks and over 60 years of age
Family history of ovarian or bowel cancer, raised CRP/ESR

*Examination*     Weight
Hands, eyes (anaemia, jaundice), abdomen, PR (masses, blood)
+/– pelvic examination (ovarian cancer)

## Interpersonal skills

*ICE*     Precipitant – *"Has anything happened recently?"*
*Stressors*
>    Work/home/relationship

*Depression screen*     Low mood, anhedonia, anxiety

## Management

*Investigations*     FBC, coeliac screen (EMA/TTG), ESR/CRP
*Do **not** do:*
>    Ultrasound scan, TFTs, $H_2$ breath test, endoscopy, faecal tests (occult blood, ova/cysts/parasites)

*Management*   Importance of "self help" in management of IBS
*Conservative*
  Diet
  Exercise
  Relaxation and leisure – encourage patient to make time for this
  Symptom diary
*Medical*
  Antispasmodic = first-line
  TCA = second-line
*Alternative*
  Do not encourage acupuncture, reflexology, aloe vera
*Psychological*
  Only if no effect of medical treatment for 12 months
  Try CBT, hypnotherapy, psychological therapy

*Follow up*   Written info, follow up, refer, inform red flags

# Dietary advice for IBS

*Based on NICE Guidelines (2008)*

Regular meals, take time to eat, don't skip meals.

Fluids: 8 cups non-caffeine fluid a day.

Bloating – encourage oats and linseed, reduce other fibre (bread, bran).

Probiotics – try for at least 4 weeks.

Reduce:
- caffeine to 3 cups/day
- fresh fruit to 3 portions a day
- alcohol, fizzy drinks, artificial sweeteners (if diarrhoea)

# Medical treatments for IBS

*Based on NICE Guidelines (2008)*

First-line: antispasmodic

Aim for "soft well-formed stool":
- loperamide for diarrhoea
- laxatives for constipation – avoid lactulose

Second-line: TCA, amitriptyline 5–10 mg nocte (up to 30 mg) – analgesic effect
- Follow up after 4 weeks.
- SSRI only if TCA fails.

# Rectal bleeding

## Data gathering

*History* How much bleeding?
Relationship to stool (?mixed with stool ?coating stool ?only on toilet paper)
Colour of blood – ?bright red ?dark red
Melaena, any other bleeding
*Associated symptoms*
    Anal itching and/or pain
    IBD: fever, mucus
    Abdominal pain
*Risk factors for piles*
    Constipation, heavy lifting, chronic cough
*Past medical history/family history*
    Bowel cancer, bleeding disorder, ?national bowel cancer screening if >60
      years old
*Drug history*
    Aspirin, warfarin, NSAIDs

*Social history* Alcohol, smoking

*Red flags* Weight loss, change in bowel habit, persistent vomiting, >40 years of age

*Examination* Weight, BP, temperature, pulse
Anaemia, jaundice, lymphadenopathy
Abdomen, PR

## Interpersonal skills

*ICE* Vital to explore ideas and concerns

*For patient* Endoscopy: *"A small telescope with a camera put up into the back passage
to investigate cause of bleeding"*
*"Most episodes of bleeding from the back passage are mild and stop on
their own"*

## Management

*Investigations* Bloods – FBC, U&Es, LFTs, ESR

*Management* Stop NSAIDs
Refer immediately if substantial blood loss, in shock or melaena
Refer urgently for endoscopy if red flags (under 2 week rule)
Treat anal symptoms (see **Pruritus ani**)

*Safety net* Wait and see if <40 years and no red flags – follow up 4–6 weeks
Seek medical attention if red flags or recurrent

# Constipation in adults

## Data gathering

**History**    *Diet and exercise*
>>> Fruit, vegetables, fibre, oral fluid intake
>>> *Obstruction*
>>> Pain, vomiting, distension
>>> Recent/previous surgery
>>> *Genito-urinary*
>>> Difficulty passing urine
>>> *Drug history*
>>> Opiates
>>> *Family history*
>>> Bowel cancer

**Red flags**    Change in bowel habit, weight loss, bleeding, vomiting

**Examination**    Weight
>>> Anaemia, abdomen, enlarged bladder, *per rectum*

## Interpersonal skills

**ICE**    Effect on life, overflow incontinence, embarrassment

## Management

**Management**    *Conservative*
>>> Fibre – fruit, vegetables, cereals, bread
>>> Water
>>> Exercise
>>> *Medical*
>>> Movicol, senna, lactulose, glycerol supplements, microenema, phosphate enema
>>> *Surgical*
>>> Treat fissure or cause

**Safety net**    Refer if red flags

# Diarrhoea

## Data gathering

| | |
|---|---|
| *History* | *"What do you mean by diarrhoea?"* |
| | ?Frequency of stool, ?loose or watery stools, ?steatorrhoea |
| | Blood in stool |
| | *Associated symptoms* |
| |     *GI*: nausea/vomiting/haematemesis, abdominal pain, fever |
| |     *GU*: urinary symptoms, haematuria, discharge |
| | *Risk factors* |
| |     Unwell contacts |
| |     Suspicious food |
| |     Recent travel |
| |     Recent antibiotics |
| | *Past medical history/family history* |
| |     IBD, thyroid disease |
| *Social history* | Occupation, alcohol |
| *Red flags* | Dehydration, uncertain diagnosis, toxic patient, acute abdomen |
| *Examination* | BP, weight, pulse, temperature, jaundice, dehydration |
| | Abdomen |

## Interpersonal skills

| | |
|---|---|
| *ICE* | |
| *For patient* | *"Infection of digestive system"* |

## Management

| | |
|---|---|
| *Investigations* | Usually none required |
| | Faeces: ova, cysts, parasites, MCS |
| | Faecal calprotectin if considering IBD |
| | Urine: dipstick, MCS |
| | Bloods: FBC, U&E, LFTs, TFTs, coeliac screen, ESR |
| *Management* | Treat as per cause: |
| | *Gastroenteritis*: oral fluids, avoid loperamide (use for social reasons only) |
| | *Dysentery*: oral fluids, antibiotics if severe or proven |
| | *IBD/coeliac disease*: refer for specialist assessment |
| *Safety net* | Inform patient to seek attention if not resolving; blood in stools or red flags |
| | Refer urgently if dehydrated, toxic or acute abdomen |

# Pruritus ani

## Data gathering

**History**   *Threadworms*
  Worms in stool
  Peri-anal rash
*Piles*
  Heavy lifting, chronic cough, strain at stool, constipation, rectal blood, anal lumps
*Fissure*
  Pain on bowel opening
*Past medical history/family history*
  DM, psoriasis, eczema, atopy

**Examination**   Anaemia, abdominal mass, rectal mass, skin tags

## Interpersonal skills

**ICE**   Washing powders, etc.
Effect on life

## Causes

*Threadworms*: especially in children (egg deposition causes itch – treat child or whole family).

*Local*: haemorrhoids, fissures.

*Infection*: fungal (beware DM, immunosuppression).

*Skin*: psoriasis, contact dermatitis.

## Treatment

*Infections*
- Wash hands and nails after visiting toilet (prevent worms).
- Dry peri-anal area after bowel opening and keep clean.
- Avoid irritants/allergens (could be treatment cream).
- Try empirical treatments
  - Threadworms (mebendazole 100 mg stat., repeat after 2 weeks if re-infection).
  - Try hydrocortisone +/− antifungal ointment nocte.

*Fissure*
- *Conservative*: high fibre diet/lactulose to allow fissure to heal.
- *Medical*: steroid/LA suppositories before opening bowels (e.g. Scheriproct); GTN ointment relieves anal muscle spasm pain.
- *Surgical*: anal stretch, partial internal sphincterotomy.

*Haemorrhoids*
- If rectal bleeding present, ensure no red flags (see **Rectal bleeding**)
- *Conservative*: avoid constipation and straining at stool, laxative/high fibre diet (changing to wholegrain bread, pasta and rice can be very effective for mild symptoms).
- *Medical*: steroid/LA ointment or suppository.
- *Surgical*: phenol injection cures 50%; refer for haemorrhoidectomy if 3rd degree, painful++, bleeding++, failed with phenol.

# Anaemia

*Based on CKS Guidelines (2013)*

## Data gathering

*History*    *Anaemia*
> Lethargy, SOB, palpitations, chest pain

*Diet*
> Lack of red meat or green leafy vegetables

*Bleeding*
> Menorrhagia, PO/PR bleeding, melaena, haematuria, haemoptysis, epistaxis

*Gastro-intestinal symptoms*
> Change in bowel habit, indigestion, vomiting/nausea, abdominal pain

*Chronic disease*
> Renal failure, rheumatoid arthritis, IBD, cancer

*Haematology*
> Easy bruising, infections

*Past medical history/family history*
> Anaemia, sickle cell disease, thalassaemia, thyroid disease

*Social history*    Smoking
Alcoholism
Pregnancy

*Red flags*    Weight loss, bleeding, dyspepsia, angina, easy bruising, bone pain, heart failure symptoms/signs

*Examination*    BP, weight
Pallor, pale conjunctiva, koilonychia, glossitis
Heart, chest, abdomen – abdominal mass, organomegaly

## Interpersonal skills

*ICE*    Effect on life and occupation

*For patient*    *"Haemoglobin is a chemical in red blood cells which carries oxygen around the body. Anaemia means there is too little haemoglobin in the blood. There are various causes."*

## Management

| | |
|---|---|
| *Investigations* | FBC and film, vitamin B12, folate, iron studies<br>Haemoglobin electrophoresis<br>LFTs, TFTs, ESR, coeliac screen |
| *Management* | Treat cause<br>Diet, iron supplements |
| *Safety net* | If no cause found refer for investigation – usually GI tract for endoscopy<br>If Hb <7 or symptomatic refer for blood transfusion<br>Monitor FBC as per cause |

## Note

- Exclude B12 deficiency before starting folic acid to avoid precipitation peripheral neuropathy.
- B12 deficiency can cause neurological symptoms (unlike folate deficiency).

## Classify anaemia by mean cell volume

*Microcytic*: iron deficiency, haemoglobinopathies (sickle cell disease, thalassaemia).

*Normocytic*: blood loss, chronic disease, bone marrow failure, haematological disease, hypogonadism.

*Macrocytic*: vitamin B12 or folate deficiency, alcoholism, hypothyroidism.

*Also*: hereditary or haemolytic anaemias.

## Iron deficiency anaemia (CKS Guidelines 2013)

Refer urgently under 2 week rule if:
- coexisting dyspepsia at any age
- Hb <11 in man with unexplained iron deficiency anaemia (IDA) for upper and lower GI endoscopy
- Hb <10 in woman with unexplained IDA who is not menstruating for upper and lower GI endoscopy.

Patients who do not need urgent referral as above but still have unexplained IDA will need investigation with upper and lower GI endoscopy.

Treat with iron supplementation whilst awaiting investigations.

A diagnostic trial of iron supplementation should only be used in women with menorrhagia or during pregnancy.

# Liver disease

## Data gathering

*History*   Malaise, lethargy, jaundice, bleeding PO/PR
*Viral hepatitis*
    Travel, blood transfusions, sexual history, tattoos, body piercings
*Family history*
    Wilson's disease, haemochromatosis, jaundice
*Drug history*
    Including over-the-counter preparations

*Social history*   Alcohol
Recreational drugs (solvents, mushrooms)

*Red flags*   Encephalopathy

*Examination*   BMI
Well or ill
Mental state
Jaundice, signs of liver disease
Abdomen, ascites, organomegaly

## Interpersonal skills

*ICE*

*For patient*   "*Three types of liver disease due to alcohol*:
- *fatty liver*: due to a build-up of fat, reversible upon stopping drinking, no symptoms usually
- *alcoholic hepatitis*: liver inflammation in which some patients have symptoms depending on severity
- *cirrhosis*: liver tissue replaced by scar tissue, which causes irreversible damage and loss of function"

## Management

*Investigations*   FBC, U&Es, LFTs, INR/coagulation screen, glucose, ferritin, copper studies, hepatitis screen, EBV, CMV, autoantibody screen, immunoglobulins, alpha-fetoprotein, a1-antitrypsin
Ultrasound scan of liver

*Management*   Treat as per cause
Stop alcohol and hepatotoxic agents

*Safety net*   Refer as per cause
Urgent referral if acute liver failure or unwell

# Inguinal hernia

## Data gathering

| | |
|---|---|
| *History* | How noticed? |
| | Pain? Reducible? |
| | *Risk factors* |
| | Chronic cough, heavy lifting, obesity, constipation |
| *Social history* | Occupation |
| *Red flags* | Strangulation/obstruction – pain, vomiting, distension, absolute constipation (unable to pass faeces or flatus) |
| *Examination* | BMI |
| | Abdomen, both inguinal regions, external genitalia |
| | Often easier to palpate hernia when patient standing up |
| | Cough impulse, reducibility, auscultation, transillumination |

## Interpersonal skills

| | |
|---|---|
| *ICE* | Effect on life, concerns |
| | Check patient's understanding of what a hernia is |
| *For patient* | *"Contents of abdomen protrude through weakness in abdominal wall"* |

## Management

| | |
|---|---|
| *Investigations* | Ultrasound scan |
| *Management* | *Conservative* |
| | Avoid precipitant, e.g. straining |
| | Weight loss |
| | Watch and wait: |
| | • especially if not fit for surgery |
| | • hernia can enlarge with time |
| | • explain risk strangulation/obstruction |
| | • can use truss to keep hernia in place |
| | *Surgical* |
| | Especially if young or gives history of episodic strangulation |
| *Safety net* | Warn patient about symptoms of obstruction |
| | Needs hospital admission if obstructed |

# Coeliac disease

*Based on NICE Guidelines (2009)*

## Data gathering

| | |
|---|---|
| *History* | *Symptoms* |
| | GI: diarrhoea, nausea, vomiting, abdominal pain, bloating |
| | General: fatigue, TATT, weight loss, failure to thrive |
| | Has patient noticed gluten-containing foods bringing on symptoms? |
| | *Diet* |
| | *Associated conditions* |
| | Autoimmune conditions, IBS, T1DM |
| | Down syndrome, epilepsy, osteoporosis |
| | Recurrent miscarriage, subfertility |
| | *Family history* |
| *Social history* | |
| *Red flags* | |
| *Examination* | General: BMI, short stature, anaemia |
| | Sore tongue |
| | Hair thinning |
| | Abdominal distension |

## Interpersonal skills

| | |
|---|---|
| *ICE* | |
| *For patient* | *"Caused by reaction of the bowels to gluten which is found mainly in wheat, barley and rye."* |
| | *"Treatment is with a gluten-free diet"* |
| | *"If blood test is positive, we will need to confirm diagnosis with a biopsy"* |
| | *"Blood test only accurate if you continue to eat gluten-containing diet"* |
| | *"Should eat gluten in >1 meal every day for 6/52 before testing"* |
| | *"Should not start gluten-free diet until diagnosis confirmed on biopsy"* |
| | Explain implications of positive coeliac test to family members |

## Management

| | |
|---|---|
| *Investigations* | Stool sample: rule out infective diarrhoea |
| | FBC, LFTs, ESR, calcium in all cases |

Serological testing to see if further investigation required
Self-testing is not a substitute for formal diagnosis
Diagnosed with intestinal biopsy (specialist referral)

*Management*   Lifelong gluten-free diet (no wheat, barley, rye +/– some oats)
Patient is eligible for a restricted supply of gluten-free foods on prescription
Yearly pneumococcal vaccination (hyposplenism)
Dietician
May require initial supplements: iron, folate, calcium
Pre-conception females: folic acid 5 µg OD

*Safety net*

# Summary of NICE Guidelines (2009) on coeliac disease

*Delayed diagnosis and treatment can result in:*

- continuing symptoms
- complications:
  - osteoporosis and increased fracture risk
  - complications in pregnancy, subfertility
  - increased risk of GI malignancy
  - growth failure, delayed puberty
  - dental problems

*If patient unable/unwilling to reintroduce gluten into their diet before testing then:*

- refer to GI specialist
- inform patient that it may be difficult to confirm diagnosis and may have implications for prescribing gluten-free foods

*Serological testing*

- IgA tissue transglutaminase (tTGA) = first-line.
- IgA endomysial antibodies (EMA) = second-line, use if tTGA is equivocal.
- Anti-gliadin antibodies (AGA) should no longer be used.

# Diabetic review

## Data gathering

*Symptoms*   "How have you been?"
1. Energy levels
2. Polydipsia/polyuria
3. Recurrent infections – skin, genito-urinary, respiratory

*Diabetic complications*
Vision
Sensory disturbance, weakness
Sexual functioning
Chest pain, SOB

*Monitoring*
Home blood sugar measurements
Medication review: compliance with treatment

*Social history*   Smoking, alcohol, drugs, diet, exercise
Depression and anxiety screen
Driving
Occupation

*Red flags*   DKA: vomiting, confusion, DIB
HONK: extreme thirst, polyuria, drowsiness, nausea, high/low blood sugars

*Examination*   BMI, BP, waist circumference, urine dip
Visual acuity and retinal screening
Peripheral neuropathy – reflexes, sensation
Peripheral pulses
Foot care – infections, ulceration, footwear

## Interpersonal skills

*ICE*   Systematic exploration of patient's symptoms; ICE early in consultation
Medication compliance – if not, why not?
Depression and anxiety screen
Consider checking patient understands difference between blood glucose and HbA1c

*For patient*   "Everyone has small amount of sugar in their blood. In diabetes blood sugar (glucose) is too high. This is due to lack of effectiveness of a hormone called insulin which is made by the pancreas"

> *"Whenever you eat, it causes your blood sugar to go up. This is because sugar from the food you eat goes into your digestive system and is absorbed into the bloodstream"*
>
> *"How well do you think your diabetes is being controlled?"*
>
> *"What do you think prevents you from better controlling your diabetes?"*
>
> *"Stopping smoking, regular exercise and a healthy diet can stop diabetes getting worse, and prevent its complications"*
>
> *"The HbA1c allows us to see how well your diabetes is being controlled over a 3–4 month period"*
>
> *"Long term high blood sugar can cause damage to kidneys and eyes and can cause heart disease"*

# Management

**Investigations**  Urine – microalbuminuria, ACR, ketones
Bloods – FBC, U&Es, glucose, HbA1c, lipids
Screening – retinal screening, foot ulcers

**Management**  *Conservative*
Structured education programmes, support groups
Diet, weight optimisation, smoking cessation
Exercise – aim for 30 mins five times a week
Patient may need to inform DVLA, free prescriptions
*Medical*
Metformin/sulphonylureas: start if HbA1c >48 mmol/mol (6.5%) despite lifstyle advice
Warn regarding hypoglycaemia if starting sulphonylurea
*Prevention of complications*
Cardiovascular: statin, control BP, ?aspirin
Renal: ACE inhibitor if microalbuminuria
Foot: annual podiatry if at risk
Depression screen
Immunisations: flu, pneumococcal

**Safety net**  Refer to A&E if HONK or DKA
Repeat HbA1c and regular review 2–6 monthly
Consider referring to DM clinic for insulin therapy initiation if HbA1c >7.5% despite treatments in primary care

# Type 2 diabetes mellitus

*Summary of NICE Guidelines (2010)\* and SIGN Guidelines (2011)\*\**

## Diagnosis (WHO criteria)

Based on symptoms and biochemistry:
- <u>Symptoms:</u> polyuria, polydipsia, weight loss
- <u>Biochemistry:</u>
  - fasting glucose ≥7.0 or
  - OGTT: glucose ≥11.1 2 hours after 75 g oral glucose load

If patient has no symptoms, repeat biochemistry tests to confirm diagnosis.

Do not use HbA1c to test for diabetes in these patients:
- with symptoms <2 months
- pregnancy or childhood/young people
- if suspecting type 1 diabetes.

## Conservative management

Patient education is central to management, ideally as part of a <u>structured, evidence-based group education programme.</u>

Controlling cardiovascular risk factors (e.g. diet, exercise, smoking) prevents both microvascular and macrovascular conditions.

### Diet
- No specialist/specific diet for diabetics – discourage foods specifically marketed for people with diabetes.
- Tailor to patient's needs, weight loss as appropriate.
- High fibre, low fat, low glycaemic index.
- Include low fat dairy and oily fish.
- Alcohol within normal healthy limits.

### Regular exercise
- Prevents onset of diabetes.
- Aim for 30 minutes exercise 5 days a week.
- Over 65s should also aim for this, being as physically active as their abilities allow.

### Depression
- Higher incidence of depression in diabetics, even higher if complications present.
- Treating depression associated with improved glycaemic control.

### Self monitoring**

- Monitor blood glucose if on insulin.
- T2DM: no routine monitoring with blood or urinary glucose.
- Consider monitoring if:
  - high risk of hypoglycaemia
  - acute illness or fasting (e.g. Ramadan)
  - planning pregnancy or pregnant
  - significant changes in medications

## Medical management*

Start medication if HbA1c >48 mmol/mol (6.5%) despite lifestyle treatment.

Three main treatment steps:
1. Metformin; slowly increase dose to minimise side effects, monitor U&Es, LFTs.
2. Add sulphonylurea if HbA1c >48 mmol/mol (6.5%); warn regarding hypoglycaemia.
3. Add insulin if HbA1c >58 mmol/mol (7.5%) with metformin + sulphonylurea.

Other agents can be used if any of above three are not appropriate:
- Thiazolidinediones or DPP-4 inhibitors (gliptins) can be used if sulphonylurea inappropriate. Only continue if >0.5% reduction of HbA1c in 6 months.
- Sitagliptin or thiazolidinedione can be used instead of insulin.
- Exenatide instead of insulin together with metformin + sulphonylurea, especially if BMI >35. Only continue if >1% HbA1c reduction and >3% weight loss in 3 months.
- Acarbose – only if other oral agents not tolerated.
- Thiazolidinediones (glitazones) – warn regarding oedema, stop if CCF.

## HbA1c*

Set individual targets, avoid lowering to less than 48 mmol/mol (6.5%).

Monitor 2–6 monthly.

## Primary prevention of cardiovascular disease

### Blood pressure*

- Aim for BP <140/80 (or <130/80 if organ damage – CVD, eye, kidney).
- Monitor 4–6 monthly if treated stable HTN (annually if no treatment required).
- Lifestyle advice: diet, exercise, weight, low salt, etc.
- ACE inhibitor = first-line.
- CCB or thiazide diuretic = second-line.
- CCB = first-line if patient may become pregnant
- Consider starting two treatments initially if Afro-Caribbean.
- Avoid alpha and beta blockers in diabetics**.

### Blood lipids

- Diet and lifestyle.
- Annual review of weight and CVD risk.
- Offer simvastatin 40 mg for all T2DM patients aged over 40 regardless of baseline cholesterol**.
- Fibrate if raised triglycerides not controlled with lifestyle or statin*.
- Aim for total cholesterol <4.0 and LDL <2.0*.
- Increase simvastatin to 80 mg or another statin or ezetimibe if target not reached*.
- Do not routinely use nicotinic acid or omega-3 fish oils*.

### Aspirin

At the time of writing there is no consensus on when aspirin should be prescribed in diabetics. Here is what NICE, SIGN and MHRA have to say:

- NICE: aspirin if >50 years or raised CVD risk and BP <145/80
- SIGN: aspirin not recommended for primary prevention of cardiovascular disease in diabetics
- MHRA: Aspirin is not licensed for primary prevention of vascular events

# Diabetic nephropathy

Annual screening with urine ACR, serum creatinine, eGFR.

### Microalbuminuria

- Earliest sign of DM nephropathy.
- ACR >2.5 in men or 3.5 in women.
- Predictor of mortality, CVD mortality and morbidity, end stage renal disease.

### Diabetic nephropathy

- >300 mg albumin/day in urine.
- Stronger predictor of mortality, CVD mortality, end stage renal disease.
- May exist with normal creatinine.

### Management

- Reduce BP as much as possible; this reduces GFR and proteinuria.
- ACEi = first-line, regardless of BP, titrate to maximum dose.
- ARB if ACEi not tolerated.
- Protein restriction diet not recommended in early renal disease.
- Screen annually for anaemia (may need erythropoeitin treatment).

# Diabetic eye disease

Annual retinal screening with digital retinal photography and visual acuity testing.

To prevent onset and progression:

- HbA1c at 53 mmol/mol (7%) = ideal
- BP <130/80

Specific treatments = laser photocoagulation, vitrectomy, cataract extraction.

If visually impaired: community support, low vision aids, maximise benefits.

Refer if maculopathy, pre-proliferative retinopathy, unexplained reduction visual acuity.

# Diabetic foot complications

- Prompt antibiotics for infections (local policies).
- Annual foot screening and education for low risk.
- Refer to specialist diabetic foot service if active foot complications.
- Annual podiatry if previous diabetic foot disease, loss of sensation, PVD or high risk.

### Neuropathic pain (NICE 2013)

- Offer either tricyclic (unlicensed), duloxetine, pregabalin or gabapentin.
- If one of the above 4 do not work, each of the remaining 3 can be tried.
- Short-term tramadol for breakthrough pain only.
- Capsaicin cream can be used for localised symptoms if patient does not want or cannot tolerate oral treatments.

### Gastroparesis

- Trial of metoclopramine, domperidone, erythromycin.

### Erectile dysfunction

- Review annually.
- Offer Viagra/Cialis if no CIs.

# Gestational diabetes

*Summary of NICE Guidelines (2008) and SIGN Guidelines (2011)*

Screening should be offered to all pregnant women.

## Diagnosis

OGTT using different values (fasting glucose ≥5.1, 1 hr ≥10, 2 hr ≥8.5).
Do not use HbA1c for diagnosing GDM.

## Risk factors

- Obesity (BMI >30).
- Previous gestational DM.
- Previous macrosomic baby (>4.5 kg).
- Family history/ethnicity (Black Caribbean, South Asian, Middle Eastern).

## In T1DM

- Pregnancy should be planned with multidisciplinary team.
- Importance of contraception/family planning services.

### T1DM gives increased risk of:

- DM complications: ketoacidosis, hypoglycaemia, microvascular complications
- Obstetric complications: miscarriage, infection, pre-eclampsia, premature labour
- Foetal complications: malformations, distress, hypoglycaemia, intrauterine death

### Planning for pregnancy in T1DM

- Maintain normal (non-diabetic) blood glucose as much as possible.
- High dose folate up to week 12/40.
- Offer preconception HbA1c, aim for <43 mmol/mol (6.1%).
- Retinal examination: before pregnancy, during each trimester.
- Stop oral hypoglycaemic agents except metformin during pregnancy.
- Stop statins, ACEi and ARB during pregnancy.
- Consider starting insulin.

## Management

- Diet, weight, exercise.
- Specialist input.
- Monitoring: blood glucose, urinary ketones (ketoacidosis).
- Early viability scan, detailed anomaly scan at 20–22/40.
- Delivery at consultant-led maternity unit.
- Early breastfeeding to avoid neonatal hypoglycaemia.
- Follow up after pregnancy to ensure no progression to T2DM.

# Goitre

## Data gathering

| | |
|---|---|
| *History* | How first noticed, time-course |
| | Recent illness, pregnancy |
| | Effect on breathing, swallowing |
| | *Diet* |
| |     Iodine deficiency (dairy products, iodised table salt, seaweed) |
| | *Hyperthyroidism*: weight loss, anxiety, tremor, palpitations, menstrual disturbance |
| | *Hypothyroidism*: weight gain, lethargy, hoarse voice, dry skin, constipation, menstrual disturbance |
| | *Family history* |
| |     Thyroid disease, autoimmune conditions including diabetes |
| *Social history* | Smoking, diet |
| *Red flags* | Thyrotoxic crisis: fever, agitation, confusion, heart failure, unwell patient |
| *Examination* | Midline swelling, moves with swallowing |
| | Retrosternal extension, thyroid bruit (moves with tongue protrusion only = thyroglossal cyst) |
| | Neck, eyes, pulse, tremor, skin/hair |
| | Proximal myopathy, reflexes |
| | Mental state |

## Interpersonal skills

| | |
|---|---|
| *ICE* | Effect on life |
| *For patient* | "*Gland at base of neck that makes a hormone called thyroxine. This thyroid hormone keeps the body functioning (metabolism) at the correct rate*" |

## Management

| | |
|---|---|
| *Investigations* | Bloods – TFTs, thyroid auto-antibodies |
| | USS thyroid |
| *Management* | *Hyperthyroidism* |
| |     Refer all cases for specialist diagnosis |
| |     Consider propranolol if tremor or tachycardia to prevent AF |
| |     Cambimazole or propylthiouracil only under specialist advice |
| |     May need radioactive iodine therapy or surgery |

*Hypothyroidism*
> Refer if young or unwell
> Oral levothyroxine replacement titrated against 1–3 monthly TFTs
> Ensure TSH not suppressed to avoid risk of osteoporosis

*Safety net*   Urgent referral if thyrotoxic crisis (mortality 10%)

# Carbimazole

- Should be initiated under specialist advice.
- Warn patient that they need to seek medical attention if signs of agranulocytosis, e.g. sore throat, fever.

# Tired all the time

## Data gathering

| | |
|---|---|
| *Clarify symptoms* | *"What do you mean by tiredness?"* (physical, mental, malaise) |
| | *"When are you tired? How long has it been going on for?"* |
| | *Ideas* |
| | Ask early on about ideas |
| | *Sleeping habits* |
| | When does the patient go to bed? When do they wake up? |
| | OSA: daytime napping? Difficulty sleeping? Refreshed when they wake up? |
| | *Medical causes (in 20–30% of cases)* |
| | Recent illness? Weight loss? |
| | Other symptoms? e.g. gastro-intestinal symptoms, exercise, SOB |
| | Diabetes: polyuria, polydipsia |
| | Thyroid disease |
| | *Psychological causes (in 50% of cases)* |
| | Depression/stress/anxiety |
| | *Past medical history/family history* |
| | Autoimmune conditions, malignancies, neurological |
| | *Drug history* |
| | Herbal/OTC, sedatives |
| *Social history* | Alcohol, drugs, smoking, caffeine |
| *Red flags* | Unexplained weight loss, bleeding, night sweats, pains |
| *Examination* | Anaemia |
| | Thyroid disease |
| | Consider depression screening questions |

## Interpersonal skills

| | |
|---|---|
| *ICE* | Ask early on about ideas using open questions |
| | *Effect on life* |
| | Work, home, relationship, social network |
| | Driving, heavy machinery, care of children |

## Management

| | |
|---|---|
| *Investigations* | Urine dip for glucose |
| | FBC, TFTs, ESR, coeliac screen, vitamin D, monospot |
| | Consider CXR – TB, lung cancer |

*Management*    Sleep hygiene
Exercise
Avoid caffeine and alcohol
Treat cause

*Safety net*

# Sleep hygiene

- Bedroom for sleep and sex only.
- Wake up same time each day.
- Avoid napping during day.
- Increase daytime exercise.
- Reduce caffeine and alcohol.
- Reduce stimulation before sleep.

# Thyroid disease

| **Hypothyroidism** | **Hyperthyroidism** |
| --- | --- |
| Weight gain | Weight loss |
| Lethargy | Anxiety |
| Hoarse voice | Tremor |
| Dry skin + hair | Palpitations |
| Constipation | Irritability |
| Menstrual disturbance | Lethargy |
| | Menstrual disturbance |

## Thyroid examination

Neck, eyes, pulse, tremor, proximal myopathy, reflexes, skin/hair, +/– mental state.

*For the patient*     *"The thyroid is a gland at base of neck that makes a hormone called thyroxine. This thyroid hormone keeps the body's metabolism functioning at the correct rate"*

*"In hypothyroidism the thyroid gland doesn't produce enough thyroxine which causes the body's functions to slow down. It is important that this is treated to avoid complications such as heart disease."*

*"After starting on thyroxine tablets you will need to have regular blood tests (1–3 monthly) to monitor its levels"*

*"In hyperthyroidism there is an overactive thyroid gland which produces too much thyroxine. The outlook is good with treatment."*

# Chronic fatigue syndrome

*Based on NICE Guidelines (2007)*

Also known as myalgic encephalomyelitis (ME).

## Data gathering

*Key features*    4 month history of:
- new onset fatigue
- reduction in activity level
- post-exertional malaise

*Also*

Sleep disturbance, poor concentration/memory, headaches
Flu-like symptoms, muscle/joint pains

*Red flags*    Weight loss, sleep apnoea, focal neuropathy, arthritis, cardio-respiratory symptoms

*Social history*    Stress, alcohol, drugs
Depression, anxiety

*Examination*    No lymphadenopathy, no joint swelling

## Interpersonal skills

*ICE*    Effect on life
*"How does this limit the activities you do?"*
*"How often do you feel tired?"*
*"What is your sleep pattern like?"*
*"CFS is a condition causing long term fatigue, and can also cause problems with sleep, headaches and muscle pains"*

## Management

*Investigations*    Urine dip
FBC, U&Es, LFT, TFTs, glucose, ESR, CRP
Coeliac screen, calcium, creatine kinase
Ferritin (children and adolescents only)
*Do **not** do (NICE Guidelines):*
Ferritin in adults, B12, folate
Serology (HepB, EBV, CMV)

*Management*     Cautious optimism: "*Most people will improve*"

"*We do not understand the cause of CFS, although it may be triggered by a viral infection*"

"*There are no tests available to confirm CFS, and there is no known cure. Certain treatments can improve symptoms and most people will improve*"

*Conservative*
  Diet – balanced
  Sleep hygiene
  Relaxation techniques
  Introduce rest periods (limit to 30 minutes at a time)
  Encourage to continue work/education – stopping is detrimental

*Medical*
  Tricyclics for poor sleep or pain

*Social*
  Talk to family/carers
  Benefits, social support, ME support society

*Safety net*     Refer for specialist MDT assessment, graded exercise therapy, CBT if 6 months of mild symptoms or 3 months of moderate symptoms

## Specific management

- Nausea: smaller more regular meals, sipping fluids, drugs as last resort.
- Sleep: avoid daytime napping.

## Do not offer

- Unstructured exercise – can make condition worse.
- Complementary therapies.
- Vitamin supplements.

# Gynaecomastia

## Data gathering

|  |  |
|---|---|
| *History* | Normally physiological, i.e. in newborn, adolescence, elderly, obesity |
|  | Duration, tenderness |
|  | Sexual function |
|  | *Past medical history* |
|  |     Liver disease, HIV |
|  | *Family history* |
|  |     Breast cancer |
|  | *Drug history* |
|  |     Digoxin, spironolactone, antipsychotics, cimetidine, anti-retrovirals |
| *Social history* | Alcohol, heroin, cannabis |
| *Red flags* | Testicular mass |
|  | Suspicious of breast cancer: rapidly enlarging, >5 cm, hard or irregular breast tissue |
| *Examination* | BMI |
|  | Is this true gynaecomastia? Symmetry |
|  | Liver disease, Cushingoid appearance, signs of hyperthyroidism |
|  | Hypogonadism – secondary sexual characteristics: hair pattern, testicle size, laryngeal size, Klinefelter's syndrome |
|  | Testicular mass/tumour |

## Interpersonal skills

|  |  |
|---|---|
| *ICE* | Self esteem, effect on life |
| *For patient* | "All men normally have small amount of breast tissue. This is enlargement of male breast tissue" |
|  | Newborn: "Due to mother's female hormones (oestrogens) still circulating in newborn. Will get better in a few weeks" |

## Management

|  |  |
|---|---|
| *Investigations* | May not need any investigations if obvious cause or physiological |
|  | Bloods: |
|  | • U&Es, LFT, TFTs |
|  | • LH/FSH, hCG, oestradiol, testosterone, prolactin |
|  | • Karyotype |

*Ultrasound scan*: testes, breast tissue
CXR
Fine needle aspiration or biopsy

**Management**   *Conservative*
     Treat cause, refer as appropriate
     Reassure if physiological
     Weight loss if obesity related
     May require psychological support
   *Surgical*
     If longstanding or fibrosis has developed

**Safety net**   Refer suspected malignancy urgently under 2 week rule

# Osteoporosis

## Data gathering

**Risk factors**   Menopause
BMI <18
Chronic disease: IBD, coeliac, type I diabetes, rheumatoid arthritis, chronic
    renal failure
*Family history*
    Menopause, hip fracture
*Drug history*
    Steroids

**Social history**   Smoking, alcohol
Weight-bearing exercise

**Red flags**   Hyperthyroidism, hyperparathyroidism, osteomalacia, hypogonadism
Falls, fragility fractures

**Examination**   BMI
Loss of height
Fracture: wrist, vertebral, hip

## Interpersonal skills

**ICE**   Medicines adherence can be an issue, especially with bisphosphonates

**For patient**   *"Thinning of bones; bones are less dense than usual"*
 *"There are no symptoms"*
 *"Leaves you more vulnerable to fracturing/breaking a bone, e.g. after
    falling"*
 *"Treatment aims to reduce the risk of a fracture/you breaking a bone"*

## Management

**Investigations**   DEXA scan
Bloods: normal FBC, ESR, TFTs, Ca, Vit D, ALP, LH/FSH, testosterone

**Prevention**
**(% fracture**
**reduction)**   Stop smoking (25%)
Reduce alcohol
Weight-bearing exercise (50%)
HRT (50%)
Consider stopping steroids

***Treatment***    *Conservative*

Calcium and vitamin D for all at risk of falls or in residential care

Analgesia and rest for vertebral fractures

*Medical*

Bisphosphonates (alendronate is first line)

SERMS (e.g. Raloxifene) – reduces vertebral fracture risk in post-menopausal women

HRT = 2nd line, early menopause

*Refer for*:
- Calcitriol/Calcitonin/Teriparatide (>65 years, high risk)
- Strontium (>75 years, high risk)

***Safety net***    Exclude red flags before treating for osteoporosis

# DEXA scan

Offer this if:
- fragility fracture <75 years
- long term steroids <65 years (especially if >7.5 mg prednisolone for 3 months)

# Bisphosphonate

"*To slow rate of bone loss*".

"*Swallow with plenty of water whilst upright on empty stomach 30 mins before breakfast*".

Daily, weekly and monthly preparations.

*Treat if:*
- T score <–2.5; or if <–1.5 and major risk factor
- steroids and fracture
- long term steroid >65 years
- fragility fracture >75 years (DEXA if 65–75 years with fracture to confirm osteoporosis)

# Carpal tunnel syndrome

## Data gathering

*Symptoms*    Tingling and pain radial 3.5 fingers
Nocturnal, relieved by shaking
Weakness

*Aetiology*    Idiopathic
Pregnancy, menopause
Repetitive use (ask about occupation), trauma
*Rheumatology*: rheumatoid arthritis, scleroderma, osteoarthritis
*Endocrinology*: acromegaly, hypothyroidism
*Infiltrative*: amyloidosis, sarcoidosis, leukaemia

*Red flags*    Consider diabetic mononeuropathy
Thenar muscle wasting = red flag – refer for decompression

*Examination*    Weight
Tinel's and Phalen's tests
Thumb abduction
Thenar muscle wasting

## Interpersonal skills

*ICE*

*For patient*    *"Pressure on (median) nerve as it runs through the carpal tunnel in the
wrist."*
*"A ligament runs across the front of the wrist. The carpal tunnel is formed by
the space between the ligament and the wrist bones"*

## Management

*Investigations*    Bloods: FBC, U&Es, TFTs, ESR, C-reactive protein, glucose
Nerve conduction studies

*Management*    *Conservative*
Rest hand, avoid precipitant
Wrist splint – some relief in up to 80%, may take up to 12 weeks to work
Acupuncture – can provide short-term relief
*Medical*
NSAIDs are no longer recommended

*Surgical*
    Steroid injection
    Carpal tunnel release

***Safety net***    Refer if wasting thenar muscles or no improvement in symptoms

# De Quervain's tenosynovitis

- Thumb extensor tenderness.
- Associated with unaccustomed activity, e.g. rose pruning.
- Radial styloid tenderness, thickened tendon sheath +/– swelling.
- Finkelstein's test: enclose thumb in a fist and flex and abduct wrist.
- *Treatment*: rest 2–4 weeks, steroid injection, surgery.

# Joint pain – a general approach

## Data gathering

| | |
|---|---|
| *History* | Acute vs. chronic |
| | Traumatic vs. spontaneous |
| | Local vs. generalised |
| | *Pain* |
| | Diurnal variation |
| | Sleep disturbance |
| | *"Have you tried anything already for the pain?"* |
| | *Other symptoms* |
| | Stiffness |
| | Fatigue, fever |
| | *Precipitant* |
| | Previous injuries |
| | Recent illness |
| *Social history* | Depression screen |
| | Occupation |
| *Red flags* | Weight loss, fever, poor range of movement, poor functioning |
| | Neurology |
| *Examination* | Joint above and below |
| | Look, feel, move, special tests |
| | Function |

## Interpersonal skills

| | |
|---|---|
| *ICE* | Effect of symptoms on daily living and occupation |

## Management

| | |
|---|---|
| *Investigations* | Bloods: FBC, ESR, urate, rheumatology screen |
| | Joint fluid for microscopy |
| | X-ray, ultrasound scan, MRI |
| *Management* | Rest, analgesia |
| | Gentle mobilisation |
| | Physiotherapy if not improving |
| *Safety net* | Refer if concerned/red flags |

## Causes

- Trauma, unaccustomed use, overuse injury (ask about occupation).
- Viral illness.
- Rheumatoid arthritis, osteoarthritis, connective tissue disorders.
- Gout.
- Polymyalgia rheumatica.
- Cancers.

# Low back pain

*Based on NICE Guidelines (2009)*

## Data gathering

**History**  Lifting, bending over, trauma
Radiation to leg
Chronic back pain: depression, carer stress, hidden agenda
*"Have you tried anything already for the pain?"*

**Social history**  Occupation, finances

**Red flags**  Age <20 or >55 years
Pain: nocturnal, thoracic
Cancer: weight loss, check past medical history
Oral steroids, HIV
*Cauda-equina syndrome*
> Bladder/bowel paralysis or incontinence, leg weakness, saddle
> paraesthesia

**Examination**  *Look*
*Feel*: tenderness, vertebral steps/alignment, sacro-iliac joints
*Move*: flexion/extension, lateral flexion, rotation
Straight leg raise + sciatic stretch test (reproduces nerve root pain)
Weakness, sensation, reflexes
  - L4/5: dorsiflexion, extensor hallucis, "walk on heels"
  - L5/S1: peroneal muscles, toe flexors, "walk on toes"
Gait

## Interpersonal skills

**ICE**  Effect on life, work, mobility
Depression screen

## Management

**Investigations**  Bloods: ESR, bone profile, PSA (in elderly men)
X-ray: ankylosing spondylitis (young), vertebral collapse, cancer (elderly)
MRI (if considering surgery or alternative diagnosis)

|  |  |
|---|---|
| *Management* | *Self-management if <6 weeks* |
|  | Reassurance |
|  | Exercise and carry on with normal activities as much as possible |
|  | Posture |
|  | *Conservative if >6 weeks* |
|  | Exercise programme |
|  | Manual therapy |
|  | Acupuncture |
|  | Combined psychological/physical treatment programme |
|  | *Medical* |
|  | Analgesia (paracetamol, NSAID; consider weak opioid) |
|  | Tricyclic antidepressants if simple analgesia not working |
|  | *Social* |
|  | Sick note, effect on occupation/life |
| *Safety net* | Review 2-weekly |
|  | Refer urgently if cauda-equina syndrome |
|  | Refer for specialist assessment if unresponsive to treatment |

# Sciatica

- Pain radiates below the knee, worsened by coughing/sneezing/laughing.

# Chronic pain

- Depression screen.
- Treatment support groups, physiotherapy, refer to orthopaedics (surgery) or rheumatology (facet joint injection).

# Summary of NICE Guidelines (2009) on low back pain

Keep diagnosis under review at all times.

Encourage self-management.

## Exclude:

- malignancy
- infection
- fracture
- cauda-equina syndrome
- ankylosing spondylitis or inflammatory condition

## Investigations

Do not offer lumbar spine X-ray.

Offer MRI:
- if considering spinal fusion surgery
- to exclude conditions listed above

## Medical treatment

- Step 1: paracetamol
- Step 2: add NSAIDs or weak opioids (codeine, dihydrocodeine)
     co-prescribe PPI with NSAIDs in all over 45 years
- Offer TCA if others insufficient, start low dose, can increase to maximum antidepressant dose
- Strong opioids: short-term if severe pain, but beware dependence (e.g. buprenopine, diamorphine, fentanyl, high-dose tramadol, oxycodone)

## Conservative treatment

For pain lasting over 6 weeks offer one of the following:
- exercise programme: maximum of 8 sessions over 12 weeks (aerobic, strengthening, stretching, posture)
- manual therapy: chiropractors, physiotherapy, osteopath (spinal manipulation, spinal mobilisation, massage)
- acupuncture: maximum of 10 sessions over 12 weeks

Consider combined physical and psychological treatment programme if above fails.

## Surgery

If conservative measures fail refer to specialist spinal surgeon for opinion on spinal fusion.

## Do not offer these treatments:

- SSRIs
- injections into back
- laser, ultrasound or TENS therapies
- lumbar support
- traction

# Knee pain

## Data gathering

*History*    Traumatic vs. non-traumatic
Previous injury
Range of movement
Fever, recent illness
*"Have you tried anything already for the pain?"*
*Meniscal damage*
    Locking/giving way – usually requires orthopaedic referral

*Social history*    Occupation
Walking/stairs/function

*Red flags*    Significant severe swelling, especially if rapid onset
Fever, polyarthropathy, urethral discharge, eye symptoms
PMH of bleeding disorder or taking anticoagulants

*Examination*    Weight, fever
*Look*: swelling, redness, effusion
*Feel*: tenderness, crepitus
*Move*: flexion/extension
Ligaments, menisci, popliteal fossa
Joint above and below: hip and ankle
Gait

## Interpersonal skills

*ICE*    Effect on life
Sensitive advice regarding choice of activity may be required

## Management

*Investigations*    Bloods: FBC, ESR, LFTs, calcium, TFTs, RhF, autoantibody screen
Fluid for microscopy
USS – eg. patella tendon tear
X-ray
MRI

*Management*    *Acute trauma*
    Refer if swelling post injury – X-ray, aspiration

If can weight bear and no swelling – RICE (rest, ice, compression, elevation)

*Chronic*
Footwear
Physiotherapy
Steroid injection
Refer arthroscopy if ligament/meniscal damage

*Chondromalacia patellae*
Analgesia, rest, physiotherapy/quadriceps exercise

*Prepatellar bursitis*
Rest, analgesia +/– aspiration
Admit if cellulitis or pus aspirated

*Osgood–Schlatter*
Tender tibial tuberosity, settles over 2–3 months

*Gout, osteoarthritis, rheumatoid arthritis*
Treat as per cause

**Safety net**

# Shoulder pain

## Data gathering

*History*    Trauma
Neck pain, neurological symptoms in upper limb
Right/left handed

*Social history*    Occupation
Effect on life
Driving

*Red flags*    Dislocation, focal neurology
Don't forget: cardiac pain, gallbladder disease, neck pain

*Examination*    Neck: look, feel, move
Abduction/adduction, flexion/extension, internal/external rotation
Neurological: power, sensation
Painful arc (60–120°) = supraspinatus/rotator cuff problem

## Interpersonal skills

*ICE*    Effect on life – often affects dressing, driving, lifting, work
Who lives at home, ?coping at home

## Management

*Investigations*    Shoulder X-ray
Ultrasound scan/MRI

*Management*    Analgesia
Gentle mobilisation
Physiotherapy
Joint injection

*Safety net*    Refer if suspect fracture, dislocation or nerve damage

*Tendonitis*: associated with repeated use, settles in 2 weeks, steroid injection.

*Rotator cuff tear*: suspect if recurrent impingement, refer orthopaedics.

*Frozen shoulder*: global limitation of movement, NSAID, physiotherapy, injection, can take months or years to resolve.

*Osteoarthritis*: imaging to rule out other pathology.

*Chronic pain*: ultrasound scan, bloods (urate, ESR...), refer for specialist assessment.

# Polymyalgia rheumatica

## Data gathering

| | |
|---|---|
| *History* | Shoulder pain and stiffness |
| | Symmetrical, worse in mornings |
| | Hip pain |
| *Social history* | Brushing teeth, combing hair, eating and drinking |
| | Occupation |
| *Red flags* | Temporal arteritis: visual loss, temporal headache/tenderness, pain in jaw when chewing |
| *Examination* | 1 in 3 have temporal arteritis |
| | Decreased range of movement shoulders +/– hips |
| | Muscular tenderness |

## Interpersonal skills

| | |
|---|---|
| *ICE* | Effect on life |
| *For patient* | *"Pain and soreness caused by inflammation of large muscles"* |
| | *"Treatment is with a medication called prednisolone and will often need to be continued for 1–2 years"* |

## Management

| | |
|---|---|
| *Investigations* | Bloods: ESR, TFTs |
| *Management* | Prednisolone orally, steroid card for patient to carry |
| | Osteoporosis prophylaxis as appropriate |
| *Safety net* | Urgent ophthalmology referral if suspected temporal arteritis to prevent blindness |

# Neck pain

## Data gathering

| | |
|---|---|
| *History* | Acute vs. chronic |
| | Trauma |
| | Headache, fever, rash |
| *Social history* | Occupation, stress |
| *Red flags* | Neurological symptoms: legs and arms |
| | Meningitis |
| *Examination* | Neck, shoulder |
| | Arms and legs if neurological symptoms |

## Interpersonal skills

| | |
|---|---|
| *ICE* | Effect on life, sleep and occupation |

## Management

| | |
|---|---|
| *Investigations* | C-spine X-ray |
| *Management* | *Conservative* |
| |    Gentle mobilisation |
| |    Wait and see, physiotherapy |
| | *Medical* |
| |    Analgesia, diazepam |
| *Safety net* | Refer if neurological features |

# Rheumatoid arthritis

*Based on NICE Guidelines (2009)*

## Data gathering

| | |
|---|---|
| *History* | Unexplained persistent synovitis |
| | Often worse in the mornings with muscle stiffness |
| | Symmetrical, small joints of hands/feet |
| | *Complications* |
| |     Vasculitis |
| |     Spine, lung and eye involvement |
| | *Co-morbidities* |
| |     HTN, IHD, osteoporosis |
| |     Depression screen |

*Social history*

| | |
|---|---|
| *Red flags* | Septic arthritis |
| | Cervical myelopathy |

*Examination*

## Interpersonal skills

| | |
|---|---|
| *ICE* | Effect on life and functioning (dressing, shopping, cooking, work) |
| | Depression screen |
| *For patient* | *"Arthritis means inflammation of joints. Rheumatoid arthritis is a type of arthritis"* |
| | *"It is an autoimmune condition, which means that it's caused by our own immune system attacking parts of our body – in this case the joints"* |
| | Ensure patient knows how to access specialist care if flare-ups occur |

## Management

| | |
|---|---|
| *Investigations* | Anti-CCP, RhF |
| | CRP to monitor disease |
| *Management* | Specialist multidisciplinary team to initiate and oversee treatment |
| | *Conservative* |
| |     TENS, wax baths |
| |     Exercise |

OT, physiotherapy
Podiatry/footwear
*Medical*
Combination DMARDs (methotrexate + another DMARD + short
course glucocorticoid) within 3 months of diagnosis
Glucocorticoids for flares
NSAID/COX-2i for symptoms
*Surgical*
Surgery for deformity, pain, loss of function

***Safety net***    Annual review
Refer early for newly presenting symptoms (see below)

[**Note**] RA is a risk factor for CVD and used as part of QRISK2 scoring, therefore give CVD primary prevention as usual, e.g. Mediterranean diet, smoking cessation.

Refer urgently if (even with normal CRP/ESR/Anti-CCP/RhF):
- small joints of hands/feet affected
- more than one joint affected
- 3 months has elapsed since symptoms began

# Medical treatment

- Drug monitoring.
- Step down DMARD doses once disease controlled/stable.

# Surgery

- For deformity, pain, loss of function.
- Tendon rupture, nerve compression, stress fracture.
- Septic arthritis.

# Osteoarthritis

*Based on NICE Guidelines (2014)*

## Data gathering

| | |
|---|---|
| *History* | Pain – diurnal variation |
| | Stiffness, precipitant, locking/giving way |
| | Current treatment |
| | Effect on sleep |
| | Depression screen |
| | Falls assessment |
| *Social history* | Occupation, family life |
| *Red flags* | Septic arthritis, rheumatoid arthritis |
| *Examination* | Deformity, skin (psoriasis) |
| | Range of movement, crepitus |
| | Function, gait |

## Interpersonal skills

| | |
|---|---|
| *ICE* | Effect on life, coping at home, carer |
| *For patient* | *"Arthritis means inflammation of joints. Osteoarthritis is the most common type of arthritis."* |
| | *"Wear and tear of joints."* |
| | *"Cartilage becomes damaged and worn"* |

## Management

| | |
|---|---|
| *Investigations* | Bloods: normal FBC, ESR, urate, rheumatology screen |
| | X-ray |
| *Management* | Three core treatments: |

- weight loss
- exercise – aerobic and muscle strengthening
- footwear

*Conservative*

Heat/cold pads

TENS

Physiotherapy/occupational therapy/walking and other aids

Benefits

*Medical*
    Paracetamol = 1st line
    Topical NSAID for hand or knee OA
    NSAID/COX2 inhibitor – prescribe with proton pump inhibitor
    Topical capsaicin
*Surgical*
    Steroid injections
    Early referral for symptoms affecting life – joint replacement
    Knee arthroscopy only for locking

**Safety net**

# Gout

## Data gathering

| | |
|---|---|
| *History* | Pain |
| | Precipitant, e.g. red meat, alcohol |
| | *Drug history* |
| | Thiazide diuretics, aspirin |
| *Social history* | Alcohol, diet |
| *Red flags* | Fever, polyarthropathy, alternative diagnosis |
| *Examination* | Gouty tophi – ears, tendons |
| | Red and inflamed joint |

## Interpersonal skills

| | |
|---|---|
| *ICE* | Effect on life |
| *For patient* | *"Type of arthritis caused by build up of substance in blood called uric acid"* |

## Management

| | |
|---|---|
| *Investigations* | Bloods: uric acid, U&Es, lipids |
| | Joint aspiration |
| *Management* | *Conservative* |
| | Reduce alcohol, weight loss |
| | Diet (avoid red meat, fizzy drinks, pulses, oily fish), oral fluids |
| | *Medical* |
| | Stop thiazide/aspirin |
| | Acute attack: NSAID (e.g. Indometacin) or colchicine |
| | Prophylaxis: allopurinol |
| *Safety net* | Refer to rheumatology if no improvement |

# Tennis elbow

## Data gathering

| | |
|---|---|
| *History* | = Lateral epicondylitis |
| | Usually unilateral |
| | Trauma, repetitive movements, unaccustomed activity |
| | Effect on life, e.g. difficulty opening jar |
| *Social history* | Occupation, support at home |
| | Driving |
| *Red flags* | Septic arthritis, neurological symptoms/signs |
| *Examination* | Both arms: exclude deformity/swelling/temperature |
| | Active and passive movements: extension/flexion, supination/pronation |
| | Sensation and power |
| | *Tennis elbow* |
| |     Tenderness at lateral epicondyle |
| |     Pain maximal on resisted wrist extension |

## Interpersonal skills

| | |
|---|---|
| *ICE* | Effect on daily life |
| | Diagnosis is usually straightforward, so targeted history and examination are required to have time to explain diagnosis and involve patient in management plan |
| *For patient* | *"Soft tissue inflammation of tendons on outside of elbow"* |

## Management

| | |
|---|---|
| *Investigations* | None required |
| *Management* | Reassurance and explanation that this is self-limiting and resolves without treatment in most cases |
| | Recovery can take several weeks to months |
| | *Conservative* |
| |     Rest, ice, avoid trigger movements |
| |     Physiotherapy |
| | *Medical* |
| |     NSAID |

*Surgical*
Steroid/local anaesthetic injection
Surgical release
*Social*
Advice regarding safe driving
Manage possible effect on occupation

**Safety net**     Consider alternative diagnosis if atypical history
EMG or referral as appropriate if neurological features

# Golfer's elbow (medial epicondylitis)

- Similar self-limiting condition with management as above.
- Occasionally associated with ulnar neuropathy.

# Raynaud's phenomenon

## Data gathering

*History*  Characteristic history of fingers/toes changing colour:
White, Blue, then Crimson (red) (remember: WBC)
Triggers: cold, emotion
Age at onset
*Past medical history/family history*
    Connective tissue disease (SLE, scleroderma), Raynaud's
*Drug history*
    Beta blockers, COCP

*Social history*  Occupation history: work with vibrating tools or in cold weather
Smoking

*Red flags*  Neurological symptoms, connective tissue disease
Underlying malignancy – rare

*Examination*  BP in both arms
Upper limb pulses
Digital ulceration

## Interpersonal skills

*ICE*  Concerns, effect on life

*For patient*  *"Due to narrowing of blood vessels in response to a trigger, usually cold
weather"*

## Management

*Investigations*  Bloods: FBC, U&Es, LFT, TFTs, ESR, rheumatological screen
    (RhF, autoantibodies)

*Management*  Treat underlying cause if found (most cases are idiopathic)
*Conservative*
    Conservative measures usually suffice
    Avoid precipitant: keep warm, gloves, consider change of occupation
    Smoking cessation, exercise
*Medical*
    Fish oil, evening primrose oil
    Nifedipine, alpha blockers, ACE inhibitors

*Surgical*
      Sympathectomy – last resort for severe symptoms

**Safety net**    Refer if underlying condition found

Features suggestive of underlying cause: unilateral, onset >30 years, male, digital ulceration.

# Dupuytren's contracture

## Data gathering

*History*   Unilateral vs. bilateral, hands vs. feet
Age at onset, how quickly progressed
Normally painless
History of trauma and manual labour
*Past medical history/family history*
Diabetes, high cholesterol, hypothyroidism, HIV
Dupuytren's contracture
*Drug history*
Anticonvulsant medication

*Social history*   Smoking, alcohol
Occupation

*Red flags*   Sarcoma in young patient – very rare

*Examination*   Little and ring fingers most often affected
Thickening of palmar fascia
Table-top test – can patient place hand flat on to a flat surface?
Measure contracture at metacarpo-phalangeal joints (MCPJ)

## Interpersonal skills

*ICE*   Effect on daily life?
Is patient right or left handed?
Patient's expectations from consultation?
Opportunity to discuss shared management plan

*For patient*   *"Fingers bend slowly into the palm of hand"*
*"Due to thickening of connective tissue in palm of hand"*
*"Not a dangerous condition"*

## Management

*Investigations*   Bloods: LFTs, TFTs, cholesterol, glucose

*Management*   Consider treating any cause
*Conservative*
Often no treatment required if mild

*Surgical*
> Usually once flexion greater than 30 degrees at MCPJ or affecting life
> One hand operated on at a time
> Warn about possible recurrence
Most non-surgical methods have very poor results

**Safety net**

[**Note**]
- link with Peyronie's disease (penile fibromatosis)
- often idiopathic
- patient usually over 50 years at presentation

# Headache

*Based on NICE Guidelines (2014)*

## Data gathering

**History**    Pain score
*Eye strain* – spectacles, vision
*Meningism* – fever, neck stiffness, rash, photophobia
*Raised ICP* – worse in morning/coughing/sneezing, vomiting, drowsiness
*URTI* – associated URTI
*Tension* – stress, dehydration/fluid intake
*Drug history*
    Codeine, CCBs, medication overuse

**Social history**    Stress at work, home, finances...

**Red flags**    Sudden onset, severe pain, worsening, >50 years at onset
Focal neurology, meningism, reduced GCS, change in personality, head
    injury, tender temporal arteries

**Examination**    BP, fundi
Temporal arteries
Neck for muscles and movements
Neuro.

## Interpersonal skills

**ICE**    Depression, stress

## Management

**Investigations**    MRI if ?underlying brain pathology (do not refer solely for reassurance)

**Management**    Headache diary
Treat cause

**Safety net**    Refer if serious features
Offer follow up

*Tension headache*:
    Symptoms:    frontal band-like headache, bilateral, squeezing or pressure, resolves
        after a few hours
    Rx:    reassurance, relaxation, exercise, paracetamol/NSAID +/– acupuncture;
        avoid opioids

*Cluster headache*:

Symptoms: severe unilateral pain around/behind eye/temple +/– eye watering or erythema/nasal watering/nasal congestion, last 30–90 mins and occur 1–2 times/day for several weeks to months

Rx: 100% oxygen, sumatriptan, prophylaxis (unlicensed: verapamil, lithium)

*Medication overuse headache:*

Rx: withdrawing overused medication – aim for 1 month without offending medication

Withdraw current medication slowly

Advise that symptoms will worsen in short-term but will then improve

May need specialist input if strong opioids are the culprit

Review in 6–8 weeks after withdrawal to confirm diagnosis

## Other causes of headache

- Migraine (see next case)
- Depression.
- Meningitis.
- Tumour.
- GCA/TA/PMR.

# Migraine

*Based on NICE Guidelines (2012)*

## Data gathering

*History*   Headache – unilateral, pulsating
Associated symptoms are fully reversible:
  • nausea, vomiting, photophobia, phonophobia
  • wanting to sleep, worse with activity
  • aura/eye symptoms
  • focal neurology: weakness/sensory disturbance, dysphasia
Triggers factors, e.g. caffeine, chocolate, red wine, cheese, alcohol, stress, fatigue
Variation with menses (treat with frovatriptan or zolmitriptan)
*Drug history*
  COCP, analgesia

*Social history*   Smoking, alcohol, stress, sleep
Occupation

*Red flags*   Patient taking COCP and migraine with focal aura or worsening migraines
  (increased risk of stroke and contraindications to COCP)
*See also* **Headache**

*Examination*   BP +/– fundi
Should have no focal neurology between attacks

## Interpersonal skills

*ICE*   Effect on life, concerns
Consider depression screen
Consider medication overuse headache

*For patient*   *"A type of severe headache, often associated with nausea and sensitivity to light"*

## Management

*Investigations*   Usually none required

*Management*   *Conservative*
  Avoid triggers, relaxation, reassurance

Acupuncture can be preventative

Symptom diary

*Simple analgesia +/– antiemetic*

Oral triptan with NSAID or oral triptan with paracetamol = first-line

Triptan should be taken during headache (not aura)

Triptan can be nasal spray or SC injection if vomiting limits use of oral preparation

Stemetil, domperidone (Migraleve contains antiemetic)

Diclofenac and domperidone suppositories available

Avoid opioids due to risk of medication overuse headache

*Prophylaxis*

Propranolol or topiramate = first-line

Gabapentin or acupuncture = second-line

Riboflavin 400 mg OD may be useful for some

Other agents include amitriptyline, valproate, pizotifen

***Safety net*** Refer if uncontrolled or uncertain diagnosis

Refer for further investigation if any of the following associated symptoms: motor weakness, double vision, visual symptoms affecting only one eye, poor balance, decreased level of consciousness

Consider stopping COCP

Offer follow up

# Transient ischaemic attack

*Based on NICE Guidelines (2008) and SIGN Guidelines (2008)*

## Data gathering

| | |
|---|---|
| *History* | Vision, speech, weakness, tingling, balance |
| | Witness, time to resolve (within 24 h), warning symptoms |
| | Previous episodes |
| | *Associated symptoms* |
| | Headache, chest pain, shortness of breath, palpitations |
| | *Risk factors* |
| | Hypertension, raised cholesterol, DM, smoking, family history/past medical history |
| *Social history* | Job, driving, smoking |
| *Red flags* | Residual focal neurology |
| | >1 episode in last week |
| *Examination* | BP, weight |
| | Atrial fibrillation, anaemia, carotid bruit, heart murmurs, chest |
| | Neurological examination with cranial nerves |
| | Peripheral pulses, fundoscopy |
| | ABCD$^2$ score |

## Interpersonal skills

| | |
|---|---|
| *ICE* | Support at home |
| *For patient* | "Results from a temporary interruption of blood flow to the brain" |
| | "Important to treat as there is an increased risk of stroke" |

## Management

| | |
|---|---|
| *Investigations* | Bloods: FBC, BMI, cholesterol, TFTs, LFTs, U&Es, glucose |
| | ECG |
| | Echo, carotid Doppler, CT/MRI of brain |
| *Management* | *Conservative* |
| | Smoking cessation, alcohol reduction |
| | Diet: low salt, low fat, fruit/vegetables |
| | Weight optimisation, exercise programmes |

*Medical*
  Aspirin 300 mg initially
  Clopidogrel as long-term anti-platelet
  Statins – consider atorvastatin 80 mg
  Control hypertension: ACE inhibitor + diuretic
*Social*
  Inform DVLA

**Safety net**   Admit if >1 episode in 1 week, ABCD$^2$ score >4, AF present, patient already
         anticoagulated or focal neurology persists
         Otherwise refer to TIA clinic within 1 week
         To seek medical attention if similar symptoms, patient information leaflet
         Regular follow up

**ABCD$^2$ score**   A score of >4 signifies high risk of early CVA and should be referred urgently
         for same day assessment
         A – Age >60 years = 1 point
         B – Blood pressure >140/90 mmHg = 1 point
         C – Clinical features: unilateral weakness = 2 points; speech disturbance
            without weakness = 1 point
         D – duration of symptoms >60 minutes = 2 points; 10–59 minutes = 1 point
         D – diabetic patient = 1 point

# TIA/cerebral vascular accident – regular follow up

- Support, social services, benefits.
- DVLA.
- Depression screen.
- Speech and language therapy, occupational therapy, physiotherapy, social services.
- Annual influenza vaccination.
- Control risk factors: e.g. BP, cholesterol.

# Head injury

*Based on NICE Guidelines (2014)*

## Data gathering

| | |
|---|---|
| *History* | Mechanism and nature of injury, e.g. was patient wearing a helmet? |
| | Bleeding |
| | Headache |
| | *Past medical history* |
| |    Coagulopathy |
| | *Drug history* |
| |    Aspirin, warfarin |
| *Social history* | Alcohol, drugs |
| *Red flags* | LOC, amnesia, vomiting, drowsiness, focal neurology, post-traumatic seizure |
| | High impact, >65 years, alcoholism |
| | Consider non-accidental injury especially in child <1 year |
| *Examination* | *Neurology* |
| |    GCS, pupils, neurological examination, local injuries |
| | *Base of skull fracture* |
| |    Bruising around eyes/ears |
| |    CSF/blood from ears and nose |

## Interpersonal skills

*ICE*

## Management

| | |
|---|---|
| *Investigations* | CT head if any red flags |
| *Management* | Analgesia: paracetamol, ibuprofen (avoid opiates as you may need to assess pupil size) |
| | Responsible adult with patient for 24 hours |
| | Future prevention of cause, e.g. refer to alcohol services |
| | Avoid driving, alcohol, drugs, sedatives until fully recovered |
| | Avoid contact sports for 3 weeks after head injury |
| *Safety net* | Refer to A&E if any red flags (also, see below) |
| | Warn regarding concussion, give written information: dizziness, headaches, poor concentration, visual disturbance |

Ask responsible adult also to read written information
Patient to go to A&E if red flags develop at home
Review in 2 weeks if still symptomatic

Consider delayed presentation of *subdural haemorrhage* if: elderly, signs of alcoholism, confusion, falls, memory and balance problems.

Refer to A&E if:
- reduced GCS
- seizure post-trauma
- focal neurology
- skull fracture
- LOC
- severe and persistent headache or headache not relieved with simple analgesia
- 2 or more episodes of vomiting
- amnesia – retrograde >30 minutes or post-traumatic >5 minutes
- high risk mechanism of injury
- coagulopathy/taking anticoagulants or antiplatelets
- re-presenting – new or ongoing symptoms

# Collapse and seizures

*Based on NICE Guidelines (2010)*

## Data gathering

| | |
|---|---|
| ***History*** | Witness account |
| | *Pre-collapse* |
| |    Warning – palpitations, chest pain, sweating, faint feeling, aura |
| |    Precipitant – cough, micturition, standing, exercise |
| | *During collapse* |
| |    LOC, duration |
| |    Movements, colour, tongue biting, incontinence |
| |    Injury |
| | *Post-collapse* |
| |    Recovery |
| | *Past medical history/family history* |
| |    Epilepsy, DM, CVD, pacemaker |
| |    Sudden death |
| | *Drug history* |
| |    Antihypertensives, tricyclics, drugs that prologue QT interval |
| ***Social history*** | Occupation |
| | Alcohol, recreational drugs, smoking |
| | Driving |
| ***Red flags*** | Focal neurology, first seizure, TIA, heart failure |
| ***Examination*** | BP: lying and standing |
| | Pulse, anaemia, heart |
| | Neurological examination |

## Interpersonal skills

| | |
|---|---|
| ***ICE*** | Witness account |
| ***For patient*** | *"A seizure is caused by a disruption of the electrical activity in the brain"* |

## Management

| | |
|---|---|
| ***Investigations*** | Bloods: FBC, U&Es, glucose, TFTs |
| | ECG |
| ***Management*** | As per cause |
| | DVLA |

| | |
|---|---|
| *Safety net* | Refer first seizure urgently under 2 week rule<br>For transient loss of consciousness, refer for cardiovascular assessment within 24 h if:<br>• ECG abnormality<br>• Heart failure<br>• Precipitated by exertion<br>• FHx of sudden death and patient <40 years<br>• FHx of inherited cardiac condition<br>• New or unexplained breathlessness<br>• Cardiac murmur on examination<br>• >65 years and no prodromal symptoms |
| *Diagnose an uncomplicated faint if:* | No evidence of alternative diagnosis and 3 'P's:<br>Posture (i.e. occur whilst standing, prevented by lying down)<br>Provoking factors (e.g. pain, medical procedure)<br>Prodromal symptoms (e.g. feeling hot, sweating) |

# Falls

*Based on NICE Guidelines (2013)*

## Data gathering

| | |
|---|---|
| *History* | Falls: frequency, any witnesses, injuries<br>Vision, continence, dementia<br>Osteoporosis |
| *Social history* | Environment/home hazards<br>Daily functioning<br>Alcohol, recreational drugs |
| *Red flags* | Exclude organic cause for fall:<br>• memory of fall<br>• warning<br>• associated symptoms<br>• UTI/infection |
| *Examination* | Confusion<br>BP, pulse, cardiovascular system<br>Neurological examination: Parkinson's disease, vision<br>Observe for gait/balance problems<br>"Get up and go" test: rise from chair without using arms |

## Interpersonal skills

| | |
|---|---|
| *ICE* | Address biological, psychological and social issues<br>Fears of falling, fear of being in nursing home<br>Depression<br>Respect patient confidentiality/autonomy if family are involved |

## Management

| | |
|---|---|
| *Investigations* | Urine MCS<br>Bloods: FBC, U&Es, glucose, TFTs, vitamin D<br>ECG<br>DEXA bone density scan |
| *Management* | Physiotherapy, occupational therapy<br>Walking aids: e.g. walking stick/frame |

*Multi-disciplinary team input*
    Falls centre
    Strength and balance training
    Occupational therapy: home hazards
    Vision test
    Medication review
Give written information

**Safety net**    Regular follow up and re-assess risk

Note:

Good practice is to screen all elderly patients for falls risk.

There is no evidence brisk walking prevents falls.

# Parkinson's disease

## Data gathering

*History*   Tremor, stiffness, slow movements
Falls
Change to handwriting, speech
Can patient cope at home?
*Drug history*
Phenothiazines

*Social history*   Smoking, alcohol, recreational drugs
Social support, family, occupation
Driving

*Red flags*   Depression, anxiety, dementia, not eating
Aspiration, infections, incontinence
Focal neurology

*Examination*   Three main features:
1. tremor – resting, pill rolling, 4–6 cycles/second
2. rigidity – cogwheel
3. bradykinesia
Shuffling gait with reduced arm swing
Expressionless face, drooling
Speech – monotonous, quiet
Small handwriting (micrographia)
Glabellar tap: Parkinson's patients continue to blink
Normal power, reflexes, sensation (and coordination in early stages)

## Interpersonal skills

*ICE*   Effect on activities of daily living, carer, 3rd party account
Emphasis on holistic care

*For patient*   *"Disorder of part of brain (substantia nigra) which helps coordinate the body's movements"*
*"The disease progresses over a number of years. The main symptoms are tremor, muscle stiffness and slowing of movement"*

## Management

*Investigations*   Usually none needed in primary care for diagnosis
Bloods: TFTs

*Management*   Aim is for symptom control, not cure
*Conservative*
Refer early for multi-disciplinary team and neurological assessment and
treatment
Physiotherapy, occupational therapy, speech and language therapy,
social services
Driving safety – inform DVLA
*Medical*
Dopamine agonists: ropinirole, cabergoline
Levo-dopa
MAO inhibitors: selegiline
*Surgical*
Pallidotomy, thalamic surgery, deep brain stimulation

*Safety net*   Regular review
Ensure patient well supported, support groups
Manage red flags, refer urgently if focal neurology, or consider alternative
diagnosis

# Dementia

## Data gathering

| | |
|---|---|
| *Symptoms* | Memory, speech |
| | Personality and behaviour: e.g. aggression, sexual disinhibition |
| | History from relative/neighbour |
| | *Differential diagnoses* |
| |     Deafness, Parkinson's disease, alcohol, depression |
| | *Past medical history* |
| |     Cardiovascular disease risk |
| *Social history* | Support at home |
| | Driving |
| | Activities of daily living |
| | Smoking, alcohol, drugs |
| *Red flags* | Focal neurology, trauma, confusion/delirium, abuse |
| *Examination* | GPCOG/abbreviated mental test score: age, time, year, address, person, place, date of birth, WW2, Prime Minister, 20–1 |
| | Exclude depression |
| | Neurological examination: should be normal |
| | Mental capacity |

## Interpersonal skills

| | |
|---|---|
| *ICE* | Ability to cope at home, continence, sleep |
| | Carer and their welfare |
| | Ensure you are seeking valid consent from the patient |
| *For patient* | *"Dementia is a condition in which problems with thinking, memory and understanding develop over time. There are many different types of dementia"* |
| | *"Alzheimer's is the most common type of dementia. The exact cause is unknown"* |

## Management

| | |
|---|---|
| *Investigations* | Urine dip and MCS |
| | Bloods: FBC, U&Es, ESR, LFTs, glucose, TFTs, syphilis, B12 |
| | In-depth mental state assessment |

| | |
|---|---|
| ***Management*** | Referral: for diagnosis/CT head/treatment – preferably with relative/friend |
| | Support, social services, nursing home, district nurse, CAB |
| | Provide written information, care plan |
| | Alzheimer's Society |
| | DVLA |
| | Independent Mental Capacity Advocate (IMCA) |
| | Treat risk factors: smoking, alcohol, obesity, HTN, cholesterol |
| | Physical health review |
| | Anticholinesterase inhibitors can be used in moderate Alzheimer's under specialist care |
| ***Safety net*** | Regular review and reassessment |

# Fungal skin infections

*History*    Feet, body, nail, scalp, hair
                      *Past medical history*
                            DM, immunocompromise, HIV
                      *Drug history*
                            Steroid, antibiotics

*Examination*    If on fingernails, examine toenails
                      Whole skin ideally

*Investigations*    MCS: skin scraping, nail clippings, plucked hair
                      Send especially if considering systemic treatment

*Management*    Clean and dry
                      Skin:
                            topical: clotrimazole tds, *continue for 2 weeks after lesions resolved*
                            oral treatment if resistant
                      Scalp: systemic treatment needed
                      *Also see below*

## Ringworm

- Use imidazoles.

## Nails

- Oral terbinafine: fingernails: 6 weeks; toenails: 3 months.
- "Pulsed" oral itraconazole: 7 days, repeat after 3 weeks (2 courses for fingernails, 3 for toenails).
- Amorolfine nail lacquer: fingernails: 3–6 months; toenails: 6–12 months (until nail grows out).

## Pityriasis versicolor

- Topical: selenium sulphide shampoo used as lotion – leave 30 mins then wash off.
- Oral: fluconazole, itraconazole (**not** terbinafine).

## Candidiasis

- *Topical*: clotrimazole.
- *Oral treatment*: fluconazole.
- *Associated angular chelitis*: nystatin ointment.

## Scalp

- Systemic treatment usually needed: terbinafine or griseofulvin.

## Oral candidiasis

- Nystatin or myconazole.

## Nappy rash

- Frequent changing nappies, air dry.
- Barrier cream (e.g. Metanium), bath oils, moisturisers.
- Satellite lesions = candidiasis: Timodine cream (= nystatin + hydrocortisone 0.5%).

## Pityriasis rosea

- Not fungal, herald patch, pink macules, no treatment needed, fade 4–8 weeks, 1% hydrocortisone for itching.

## Terbinafine

- Nails and scalp.

# Acne

## Data gathering

| | |
|---|---|
| *History* | Duration, location, ?triggers |
| | *"Do you have spots anywhere else on your body?"* |
| | Effect on self-esteem |
| | Treatments already tried |
| | Contraception/pregnancy |
| | PCOS: weight gain, menstrual irregularity, hirsutism |
| | *Drug history* |
| |     Progestogen: e.g. COCP, POP, Mirena coil |
| *Social history* | Effect on social life |
| | Relationships |
| *Red flags* | Depression, severe effect on functioning |
| *Examination* | Erythema, comedones, pustules, scarring, cysts |

## Interpersonal skills

| | |
|---|---|
| *ICE* | Effect on life, ascertain health beliefs |
| | Do not dismiss patient's concerns if acne is mild – show empathy |
| | Hidden request for contraception |
| *For patient* | *"Caused by glands under the skin producing too much oil (sebum). This can block the pores and cause acne. Common in teenage years due to change in hormone levels, but can occur at any age"* |

## Management

*Investigations*

| | |
|---|---|
| *Management* | Treat early if inflammatory to prevent scarring |
| | *Conservative* |
| |     Wash twice daily with mild soap, avoid picking/scratching |
| | *Medical* |
| |     Topical: benzoyl peroxide, retinoid creams, topical antibiotics |
| |     Oral antibiotics: e.g. oxytetracycline |
| |     • inform at least 3–6 months treatment required |
| |     • if antibiotic is teratogenic, ensure female patient understands this/ uses appropriate contraception |
| |     COCP |

*Safety net*    Regular follow up
               Refer for specialist initiation of isotretinoin (Roaccutane)

# Counteracting common myths

- Acne is not caused by poor hygiene or unhealthy diet – too much washing can be detrimental.
- Picking spots does not help and can cause scarring.
- Acne is not contagious.
- Sunbeds often do not help.
- Medical treatments do work if used correctly.

# Eczema

*Based on NICE Guidelines (2007)*

## Data gathering

| | |
|---|---|
| *History* | Dry and itchy, duration, site, itch |
| | Precipitant: allergen, stress |
| | Impact on life, sleep and self-esteem |
| | *Past medical history/family history* |
| | Atopy: hayfever, asthma |
| | *Drug history* |
| | Treatments already tried |
| *Social history* | Stress: work, home, relationships |
| | Smoking, alcohol |
| | Occupation |
| *Red flags* | Secondary infection – pain, fever, erythema |
| | Child: failure to thrive, GI symptoms (consider food allergy) |
| *Examination* | Distribution: flexural, seborrhoeic, contact (necklace, watch, belt) |
| | Erythema, papules, vesicles, crusting, weeping, dry |
| | Lichenification, scarring, excoriation |
| | Cushingoid appearance |

## Interpersonal skills

| | |
|---|---|
| *ICE* | Depression screen |
| | Empathy with patient's/parent's situation |
| *For patient* | *"Sometimes called dermatitis, inflammation of skin, itchy skin condition, can flare up from time to time"* |
| | *"Controlled and not cured"* |
| | *"Child **may** grow out of it, but it occasionally persists"* |

## Management

| | |
|---|---|
| *Investigations* | Skin patch testing if contact dermatitis and unknown allergen |
| *Management* | Avoid allergens, perfumed products, detergents (e.g. gloves when washing up, non-bio detergents) |

*Medical*
    Soap substitute: e.g. aqueous cream, emulsifying ointment
    Emollients
    Topical steroids (1% hydrocortisone for face or young children)
*Severe*
    Wet wrapping over steroids/emollients if severe
    Phototherapy
    Immunosuppression: oral steroids, tacrolimus
*Infection*
    Topical: fusidic acid cream (short courses to avoid resistance)
    Oral: flucloxacillin, acyclovir (for herpes, refer same day)
*Other*
    Antihistamine for itch (not for routine use)

*Safety net*   Regular review with compliance assessment
    Refer if unresponsive/severe or suspicion of occupational or herpes
      infection

- Exclusion diets are controversial and generally only with dietician advice in children.
- Asian and Afro-Caribbeans: extensor and discoid subtypes more common.
- Complementary therapies: no good evidence base, caution against use.

# Psoriasis

*Based on SIGN Guidelines (2010) and NICE Guidelines (2012)*

## Data gathering

| | |
|---|---|
| ***History*** | Distribution, duration |
| | Joint pain, nails and hair |
| | Treatments so far |
| | Precipitants: trauma, stress, infections, drugs (lithium, beta blockers, NSAIDs, ACE inhibitors) |
| | *Family history* |
| ***Social history*** | Smoking, alcohol |
| | Stress: work, home, relationships |
| ***Red flags*** | Erythroderma, widespread pustular psoriasis ("fluid-filled spots") |
| | New arthropathy |
| | Large effect on life/work/school |
| ***Examination*** | Clinical diagnosis |
| | Well-defined scaly silvery-red plaques on extensor surfaces and scalp |
| | Koebner phenomenon |
| | Nail pitting |
| | Arthropathy (joint swelling, dactylitis, spinal pain with early morning stiffness) |

## Interpersonal skills

| | |
|---|---|
| ***ICE*** | Effect on life/work/school |
| | Self-esteem often affected |
| | Compliance with medications can be difficult – keep number of daily treatments to a minimum |
| ***For patient*** | *"Due to increased turnover of skin cells which leads to a build-up of cells on the skin's surface"* |
| | *"Not infectious/contagious, not curable, but can be controlled with treatments"* |
| | *"Exact cause unknown, strong familial component"* |
| | *"Controlling weight, stopping smoking and reducing alcohol intake <u>may</u> improve symptoms"* |
| | *"Psoriasis <u>may</u> increase risk of cardiovascular disease and diabetes"* |

# Management

*Investigations*    Skin biopsies if difficult diagnosis (refer)

*Management*    *Conservative*
        Support groups, education
        Avoid stressors/stress
        Smoking cessation, alcohol in moderation
        Exercise and weight management (BMI <25)
       *Medical*
        Emollients
        Topical corticosteroids (short-term use)
        Vitamin D analogues (well tolerated)
        Coal tar
        Dithranol (stains clothing, irritative to skin, for flexures only)
        Tazarotene gel
       *Refer for:*

- PUVA (psoralen with ultraviolet A treatment)
- oral retinoids
- immunosuppressants – methotrexate, ciclosporin
- biological therapies – adalimumab, etanercept, infliximab

*Safety net*    Follow up in 6 weeks if treatment regime altered
        Refer if uncertain diagnosis, extensive disease or topical treatment failed
           after 2–3 months
        Erythroderma/widespread pustular psoriasis requires emergency referral
        All patients suspected of having psoriatic arthritis should be referred for
           early rheumatology assessment to prevent joint damage

# Summary of SIGN and NICE Guidelines on psoriasis

### Topical treatments

Emollients (reduces scales and itch).

*For short term, intermittent use, e.g. inflammatory psoriasis:*
- potent topical steroid/vitamin D combination cream. Do not use potent steroids >8 weeks at a time

*For longer-term topical Rx, e.g. chronic stable plaque psoriasis:*
- first-line
  - vitamin D analogue (well tolerated) for 8–10 weeks at a time
- second-line
  - coal tar
  - dithranol (stains clothing, irritative to skin, for flexures only)
  - tazarotene gel

*Scalp psoriasis*
- First-line = potent steroids (short term up to 4 weeks, intermittent use).
- Emollients.
- Salicylic acid/coal tar/oil overnight to remove thick scale.

*Nail psoriasis*
- If severe refer to dermatologist

*Facial or flexural psoriasis*
- Moderate potency topical corticosteroids (short term use).
- Coal tar (intermittently).
- Tacrolimus ointment.
- Avoid irritants such as dithranol, topical retinoids.

*Guttate psoriasis*
- This is the rapid development of small papules over wide area of body.
- Try topical therapy.
- Refer early for phototherapy if not responding.

## Diagnosing psoriatic arthropathy

- Many types of presentation, can be symmetrical or asymmetrical.
- Most frequent presentation is polyarthritis, followed by oligoarthritis.
- Dactylitis ("sausage" fingers/toes).
- Inflammatory back pain (better with exercise, night pain, early morning stiffness better on waking).

## Severe psoriasis/psoriatic arthritis

- May be associated with increased risk of cardiovascular disease and diabetes.
- Requires annual review: BMI, DM screening, BP, lipids.

# Ear pain

## Data gathering

| | |
|---|---|
| *History* | Hearing, discharge, bleeding |
| | Fever, URTI, swimming |
| | Trauma, foreign body |
| | Toothache, dental problems |
| *Red flags* | Head injury, longstanding symptoms |
| *Examination* | Ear |
| | Mastoid |
| | Temporomandibular joint |
| | Skin: shingles, boil/furuncle |
| | Cranial nerves: facial nerve |

## Interpersonal skills

*ICE*

## Management

*Investigations*  Swab if discharge

*Management*  *Acute otitis media*
  Analgesia, amoxil if persists >48 h
  *"Average duration of illness is 4 days"*
*Eustacian tube dysfunction*
  Regular warm drinks +/– decongestants
  Steroid nasal spray
*Otitis externa*
  Keep dry, antibiotic ear drops/spray: otomize, sofradex
*Perforated ear drum*
  Consider amoxicillin 1 week, refer if not improving 2–6 weeks/(earlier
    if marginal)
*Boil/furuncle*
  Analgesia +/– I&D
*Temporomandibular joint*
  Analgesia, reassurance, relaxation, dental opinion if persists
*Dental*
  Analgesia, amoxicillin, dentist

*Safety net*

*Wax*: not usually painful, treat with olive oil drops 1–2 weeks, avoid cotton buds.

# Tinnitus

## Data gathering

*History*  "What do you mean?"
Ringing, buzzing, other noise
Unilateral vs. bilateral
Loud noise exposure
Head injury
Headache
Ear infections
*Ménière's*
   Hearing loss, dizziness, earache/fullness in ear, nausea
*Depression screen*
   Effect on life, sleep
*Drug history*
   Loop diuretics, aspirin, NSAIDs

*Red flags*  Unilateral, head injury, evidence of raised ICP
Suicidal ideation: chronic tinnitus is a risk factor

*Examination*  BP
Ears: otitis externa/media, wax
Mental state to rule out hallucinations

## Interpersonal skills

*ICE*  Effect on life, depression, stress
[**Note**] Patients are often worried about a brain tumour or hypertension

*For patient*  "Tinnitus is a ringing or buzzing noise that you can hear but does not come from outside your ear"
"In many cases we do not know the cause, and often it gets better by itself"
"Can be worsened by stress and anxiety"
For longer term symptoms: "There is no cure but there are ways we can make it easier to live with"

## Management

*Investigations*  FBC (anaemia can cause tinnitus)
Audiometry

*Management*   Reassurance (patients often worried about brain tumour and hypertension)
Most self-resolve

Support groups: Tinnitus Association
Tinnitus Masker: available through ENT/tinnitus clinic
Hearing aids: can sometimes help if some deafness present
Treat co-existing problems: wax, stress, otitis

*Safety net*   Refer if:
- persistent
- unilateral (urgent referral to rule out acoustic neuroma)
- Ménière's (for diagnosis = idiopathic dilation of endolymphatic spaces)

*Causes*: anaemia, head injury, drugs, noise exposure, acoustic neuroma (unilateral), Ménière's.

# Dental pain

## Data gathering

|              |                                                                                    |
|-------------:|------------------------------------------------------------------------------------|
| *History* | May present as facial, neck or ear pain |

*History*    May present as facial, neck or ear pain
Fever, swelling, discharge/unusual taste in mouth
Previous episodes
Is patient registered with dentist?
*"Have you seen a dentist?"*

*Social history*    Diet, occupation

*Red flags*

*Examination*    Teeth, lymph nodes: tap tooth/gum with tongue depressor to elicit tenderness
Examine as appropriate:
- ENT, sinuses, salivary glands including parotid
- cranial nerves
- eyes
- skin

## Interpersonal skills

*ICE*    Important to find out patient's ICE early on
Effect on life: eating, sleep

## Management

*Investigations*

*Management*    Ensure patient understands dental consultation required for proper assessment
Analgesia
Amoxicillin 5–7 days if suspect abscess or root canal infection. Add metronidazole if severe infection is suspected

*Safety net*    Dental review

# Labyrinthitis/vestibular neuronitis

## Data gathering

*History*  Light-headed vs. sensation of rotatory movement
Precipitants: head movements, lying down, stress, trauma
Recent illness/URTI
*Associated symptoms*
    Nausea/vomiting
    Ménière's: tinnitus, fullness/sensation in ear, reduced hearing
    Infection: ear, meningitis
*Drug history*
    Aminoglycosides, antihypertensives (especially beta blockers),
        anti-convulsants

*Social history*  Driving
Alcohol, recreational drugs

*Red flags*  Neurological symptoms: headache, weakness, sensory disturbance
Unilateral tinnitus and/or hearing loss: suspect acoustic neuroma

*Examination*  Should be no abnormalities except maybe some horizontal nystagmus
Targeted neurological examination:
- cranial nerves
- cerebellar signs (DANISH – <u>d</u>ysdiadocokinesis, <u>a</u>taxia, <u>n</u>ystagmus, <u>i</u>ntention tremor, <u>s</u>lurred speech, <u>h</u>ypotonia)

ENT:
- mastoid
- Hallpike manoeuvre

## Interpersonal skills

*ICE*  Effect on life, occupation, stress

*For patient*  *"Viral infection of inner ear that controls balance"*

## Management

*Investigations*  Bloods: FBC, U&Es, TFTs, glucose
Audiometry

*Management*  *Conservative*
    Reassurance not brain tumour

Will get better by itself within a few weeks

No driving

*Medical*

Vestibular suppressants: stemetil, antihistamines, domperidone

**Safety net**  *Refer if*:
- focal neurological features or suspect acoustic neuroma
- suspect Ménière's disease
- no resolution in 4–6 weeks or rapidly worsening symptoms

# Snoring

## Data gathering

| | |
|---|---|
| *History* | How often? |
| | Disturbed sleep? Apnoeas? (witness account often required) |
| | Daytime sleepiness? Irritability? |
| | *Drug history* |
| |    Sleeping tablets |
| *Social history* | Alcohol, weight gain |
| *Red flags* | |
| *Examination* | BMI |
| | Collar size (>17 associated with obstructive sleep apnoea) |
| | ENT: any obvious obstruction |
| | Chest, heart, thyroid signs |

## Interpersonal skills

| | |
|---|---|
| *ICE* | Depression screen, effect on partner and relationship with partner |
| *For patient* | *"Obstruction can be anywhere from nose to base of tongue"* |

## Management

| | |
|---|---|
| *Investigations* | TFTs |
| | Sleep studies |
| *Management* | Weight loss, exercise, smoking cessation |
| | *Conservative* |
| |    Encourage to sleep on their side |
| |    Ear plugs for partner |
| |    Nasal dilators |
| |    CPAP (mainly for obstructive sleep apnoea) |
| | *Medical* |
| |    Stop alcohol and sedatives |
| | *Surgical* |
| |    Nasal surgery: e.g. turbinate reduction, septoplasty, polypectomy |
| *Safety net* | Support patient and partner |

# Sore throat and tonsillitis

*Based on NICE Guidelines (2008) and SIGN Guidelines (2010)*

## Data gathering

| | |
|---|---|
| *History* | Confirm symptoms: fever, sputum, DIB, pain on swallowing, E&D, D&V |
| | Treatments already tried |
| | Recent illness |
| | Travel |
| | Contacts |
| | PMH: asthma, general health |
| | COCP if considering antibiotics |
| *Social history* | Effect on life, family and work/school |
| | Alcohol |
| | Smoking |
| *Red flags* | SOB, chest pain, stridor, progressive difficulty swallowing, dehydration |
| *Examination* | Temperature |
| | Rash |
| | Throat |
| | Cervical lymph nodes |
| | +/– chest, +/– abdomen (enlarged spleen/liver if suspecting glandular fever) |

## Interpersonal skills

| | |
|---|---|
| *ICE* | *"Was there anything in particular that prompted you to come in?"* |
| | Expectations of treatment |
| | Previous experiences, e.g. pneumonia or hospitalisation |
| *For patient* | *"Likely to be a viral infection. Antibiotics not effective against viruses and may cause side-effects such as diarrhoea and vomiting…"* |
| | *"Average duration of illness is 1 week"* |

## Management

*Investigations*

| | |
|---|---|
| *Management* | Oral fluids |
| | Salt water gargle |
| | Simple analgesia (caution with NSAIDs in asthmatics) |
| | +/– Difflam spray |

+/– antibiotics (<u>not</u> amoxil) – consider delayed script

Avoid alcohol

***Safety net***    Refer for I&D if quinsy

If stridor or acute respiratory distress <u>don't examine throat</u> and admit to hospital

## Summary of SIGN Guidelines (2010) on sore throat and tonsillectomy

- 50–80% of sore throats are viral.
- 1–10% of sore throats are caused by Epstein–Barr virus (glandular fever).
- Throat swabs should not be routinely taken (cannot differentiate between commensals and infection).

## Analgesia

<u>Adults</u>: ibuprofen = first-line, paracetamol = second-line.

<u>Children</u>: paracetamol = first-line, ibuprofen = second- line (avoid ibuprofen if risk of dehydration in children due to potential renal toxicity).

## Centor score

Assess likelihood of infection being bacterial. Consider antibiotics if Centor score >3. 1 point for each of:

- tonsillar exudate
- anterior cervical lymphadenopathy
- lack of cough
- fever

## Antibiotics

If prescribed, penicillin V for 10 days is a "normal" regime.

Avoid amoxil (cross-reactivity with Epstein–Barr virus causing rash).

Should <u>not</u> be used to:

- treat symptoms in sore throats
- prevent the development of rheumatic fever and acute glomerulonephritis
- prophylaxis for recurrent sore throats

Antibiotics may prevent cross-infection with GABHS in closed institutions (e.g. barracks, boarding schools) but not for routine use in community.

**Echinacea** should <u>not</u> be recommended.

# Tonsillectomy

Watchful waiting preferred in children in mild episodes of sore throat.

When in doubt regarding suitability of tonsillectomy, recommend 6/12 watchful waiting.

Consider in <u>adults and children</u> if recurrent <u>acute tonsillitis</u>:
- the episodes of acute tonsillitis prevent normal functioning
- >7 well documented, clinically significant, adequately treated episodes within 1 year, or
- 5 or more episodes in each of the previous 2 years, or
- 3 or more episodes in each of the preceding 3 years

### *Post-tonsillectomy*

Pain may worsen for 6 days following tonsillectomy.

To prevent post-operative nausea/vomiting:
- routinely use antiemetics
- routinely use NSAIDs (also analgesics)
- consider stimulation of the acupuncture point P6 routinely if unable to use antiemetics

# Painful and red eye

## Data gathering

*History*   *General*
How much pain? History of pain
Visual disturbance, discharge, photophobia
Contact lenses, spectacles
*Specific questions*
Foreign body, trauma (abrasion)
Haloes, dusk, nausea/vomiting (glaucoma)
Reading (long sightedness)
URTI (conjunctivitis, sinusitis)
Systemic symptoms (iritis/scleritis/episcleritis)
Vesicular rash (herpes simplex)
Itchy, sore, grittiness, precipitant/allergen (conjunctivitis:
allergic/infective)

*Red flags*   Sudden loss of vision
Temporal arteritis
Acute angle glaucoma
Chronic symptoms
Trauma, chemical exposure
Severe pain

*Examination*   Inspection +/− eversion of eyelid
Fluoroscein
Eye movements
Pupil reflexes
(Consider visual acuity, fields, fundoscopy)
+/− take swab
Temporal arteritis

## Interpersonal skills

*ICE*

## Management

### Investigations

*Management*   Conjunctivitis: leave or use chloramphenicol or cromoglycate/
antihistamines

Corneal abrasion: review in 2 days, give eyepad if amethocaine/local anaesthetic used

*Safety net*    Sudden visual loss – refer immediately:
- Temporal arteritis – consider prednisolone 80 mg stat
- Acute angle closure glaucoma – consider pilocarpine 4% drops every 5 mins and acetazolamide if no contraindications

Migraine – consider referral if atypical or unsure of diagnosis

- *Painful and red*: often need urgent referral: glaucoma, herpes simplex, foreign body, abrasion.
- *Painful and not red*: often seen in general practice: stress, refractive error, **beware GCA, retrobulbar neuritis**.
- *Not painful and red*: conjunctivitis, subconjunctival haemorrhage (check BP).

Temporal artery + fever = giant cell arteritis/temporal arteritis.

Cloudy cornea and pupil dilation = glaucoma.

# Prostate cancer

*Based on NICE Guidelines for suspected cancer (2005) and prostate cancer (2014)*

## Data gathering

| | |
|---|---|
| Symptoms | Polyuria, nocturia, frequency, hesitancy, terminal dribbling, dysuria |
| | Erectile dysfunction |
| | Lower back pain |
| | FHx |
| | Ethnicity (Afro-Caribbean are higher risk) |
| *Social history* | Smoking, alcohol, drugs |
| *Red flags* | Haematuria, weight loss, bone pain |
| *Targeted examination* | DRE, abdomen (enlarged bladder) |

## Interpersonal skills

*ICE and effect on daily life*

*For patient*   *"Rare if you are under 65 years old"*

## Management

*Investigations*   Urine, PSA (also see **Prostate-specific antigen** case)

*Management*   Refer under 2 week rule if:
>      DRE is suspicious for prostate cancer
>      Raised or rising PSA in elderly patient
>      Painless macroscopic haematuria
>      Microscopic haematuria and >50 years old
>      Symptomatic and raised PSA

Ensure no UTI before PSA testing (see **Prostate-specific antigen** case)

*Safety net*   Consider monitoring in primary care if low risk, e.g. with annual PSA
If PSA is borderline and patient has no symptoms, instead of referring you can repeat PSA in 1–3 months. Refer urgently if subsequent PSA is rising.

# Prostate-specific antigen

Patient should decide, after discussion with their doctor, whether to have a PSA blood test. Important to give written information. Useful patient information leaflet is here: www.cancerscreening.nhs.uk/prostate/prostate-patient-info-sheet.pdf

The patient needs to be told the following:
- prostate cancer is but one of several causes of a raised PSA (non-specific test)
- all patients with a significantly raised PSA should have a prostate biopsy
- If PSA is normal you are unlikely to have prostate cancer, but there can be false negatives and 1 in 5 men with a normal PSA will have prostate cancer
- 2 in 3 men with a raised PSA will not have cancer
- there is no conclusive evidence that detection of early prostate cancer leads to longer survival
- the test cannot distinguish between aggressive and slow-growing cancers, and may detect tumours that would not otherwise become evident in the patient's lifetime

The test is of most value in patients who are "high risk", i.e. those >70 years, Afro-Caribbeans, and those with a family history.

At the time of the test, the patient should not have:
- a UTI within the last month
- ejaculated within prior 48 hours
- a *per rectum* examination within 1 week
- a prostate biopsy within 6 weeks

Age-related PSA reference ranges:
- 50–59 years ≥3.0
- 60–69 years ≥4.0
- >70 years >5.0

Causes of raised PSA:
- acute urinary retention/catheterisation
- BPH/TURP
- old age
- prostatitis
- prostate carcinoma

# Haematuria

## Data gathering

*History*  "*Can you see blood in your urine?*"
Painful? Clots? Frothy urine?
*Confounders*
   Beetroot, rifampicin, menstruation
*Trauma*
   Including recent urological surgery
*GU symptoms*
   Irritative/UTI
   Obstructive
*Past medical history*
   Recent illness/sore throat, kidney stones
*Drug history*
   Anticoagulants

*Social history*  Occupation – chemicals, dyes
Smoking, alcohol

*Red flags*  Weight loss, malaise, anorexia, back pain
Painless macroscopic haematuria
Persistant microscopic haematuria; "*fewer than 1% have cancer*"

*Examination*  Obtain permission, chaperone
BP, abdomen, genitalia, DRE

## Interpersonal skills

*ICE*

*For patient*  "*A cystoscopy is when a thin flexible tube is passed through the tube in the penis into the bladder ... to look for sources of the bleeding*"

## Management

*Investigations*  Urine dip and MCS
Urine ACR
Bloods for U&Es if obstructive symptoms

*Management*  Treatment as UTI if painful
Analgesia

> ***Follow up***   Repeat urine dip after 1 week if treating as UTI
> Painless macroscopic haematuria: refer urgently under 2 week rule
> Refer all children with haematuria
> <u>All</u> persistent haematuria requires further investigation

[**Note**] Main differential diagnoses are UTI, renal stone, cancer, trauma.

# An approach to management of haematuria

- Exclude infection, trauma and menstruation.
- Do not assume haematuria is due to anticoagulants or anti-platelets: investigate anyway
- Can be divided into symptomatic (i.e. with LUTS) or asymptomatic haematuria as well as microscopic and macroscopic.
- No need for laboratory confirmation.
- Check U&Es and for proteinuria.
- <u>All</u> persistent haematuria requires further investigation:
  - refer urgently under 2 week rule if painless macroscopic haematuria
  - refer to urology if: macroscopic haematuria, symptomatic microscopic haematuria at any age (in which UTI has been excluded), asymptomatic microscopic haematuria aged >40 years.
  - refer to nephrology if: urological criteria not met; declining eGFR >10 ml/min over 5 years or 5 ml/min within 1 year; eGFR <30 ml/min; ACR >30; haematuria and HTN aged <40 years

# Renal tract stone

Refer urgently if:
- first presentation
- obstruction on imaging
- very painful
- reduced renal function
- infection

Otherwise:
- fluids, analgesia
- MSU, bloods (FBC, CRP, U&Es, calcium, albumin, phosphate)
- CT KUB (can often be arranged for same day)
- refer outpatients

# Erectile dysfunction

## Data gathering

**History**    *"Tell me more about this"*
*"Are you able to have erections?"*
*"Difficulty maintaining an erection?"*
Erections at night or morning? Sexual desire?
*Onset*
     Gradual vs. sudden onset
     Previously sexually active? Previous problems?
*Past medical history*
     Cardiovascular risk factors (hypertension, DM, raised cholesterol,
       obesity)
     Peripheral vascular disease/spinal injury/radiotherapy
     Trauma/spinal injury/radiotherapy
*Drug history*
     Antihypertensives, antidepressants, beta-blockers

**Social history**    Relationship – clarify who sexual activity is with: ?wife/long term regular
     partner. Is ED with all sexual partners or just some?
Work, home, finances, other stressors
Alcohol, drugs, smoking
Exercise

**Red flags**    Urinary symptoms, haematuria, prostatism, GI symptoms

**Examination**    BMI, BP
External genitalia – Peyronie's, hypospadius, testicular atrophy
DRE if >50 years

## Interpersonal skills

**ICE**    Stress, depression and anxiety
Occupation, family, finances, sleep
Explore anxiety and difficulties within and surrounding the sexual
     relationship

**For patient**    *"Often caused by poor blood flow to penis"*
*"Stress and psychological reasons can also cause or contribute towards
     this"*
*"Smoking and alcohol can contribute towards this"*

## Management

| | |
|---|---|
| *Investigations* | Bloods: glucose, cholesterol, U&Es, hormone profile (LH/FSH, testosterone, prolactin) |
| *Management* | *Conservative*<br>    Psychosexual counselling, stress management<br>    Lifestyle advice<br>*Medical*<br>    PDE5 inhibitors*<br>*Surgical*<br>    Penile injections, prostheses, vacuum devices |

## *PDE5 Inhibitors

- Examples are sildenafil (Viagra), tadalafil (Cialis), vardenafil (Levitra).
- Take 1 hour before sex.
- "*Increases blood flow to penis*".

*Contraindications*:
- nitrates, hypotension
- recent CVA/MI/unstable angina or cardiac condition in which sexual activity is contraindicated
- severe hepatic/renal dysfunction
- caution in sickle cell disease, leukaemia, multiple myeloma (priapism)

*NHS scripts can be issued if*:
- prostate cancer/radical pelvic surgery
- pelvic or spinal injury
- DM
- renal failure
- MS, spina bifida, Parkinson's disease, polio, single gene neurological disease

# Benign prostatic hyperplasia

*Based on NICE Guidelines (2010)*

## Data gathering

| | |
|---|---|
| *History* | Urinary symptoms |

*Voiding*: hesitancy, poor stream, straining, incomplete emptying, terminal dribbling

*Storage*: frequency, urgency, urge incontinence, nocturia

*Post-micturition*: post-micturition dribbling

*Infective*: fever, dysuria, urethral discharge, polydipsia, DM

*Associated symptoms*

Incontinence, bowel habit, abdominal pain, sexual function

*Medication*

Including OTC therapies

*Social history*    Fluid intake

Caffeine

Alcohol

*Red flags*    Specific: bone pain, haematuria

General: weight loss, lethargy

*Examination*    Bladder/urinary retention, kidneys

External genitalia

Rectal examination

## Interpersonal skills

*ICE*    Effect on life

*For patient*    *"The prostate is a gland, size of a chestnut, which sits at base of bladder, and surrounds the tube through which urine passes"*

*"These symptoms are common and affect up to one-third of men aged over 65 years"*

*"Without treatment, symptoms may not worsen, and sometimes they even improve over time"*

*"If symptoms do worsen, then medication and other treatments may help"*

# Management

*Investigations*   IPSS score
Urinary frequency volume chart (NICE)
Urine – dip, MSU
Bloods – U&Es, PSA, glucose, Ca
Trans-rectal USS prostate
X-ray pelvis/hips – ?metastases

*Management*   *Conservative*
   Avoid evening fluids
   Decrease caffeine and alcohol
   Bladder retraining
   Avoid constipation
   Pads/containment devices
*Medical*
   Alpha-blocker (relaxes smooth muscle) – warn postural hypotension
   Finasteride – shrinks prostate, can take 6 months to work
*Surgical*
   TURP
*Alternative*
   Saw palmetto – can be effective!

*Safety net*   Refer if:
   • raised U&Es
   • ?cancer – haematuria, abnormal PR, weight loss...
   • treatment resistant
   • urinary retention

**Think**: could urinary symptoms be due to diabetes?

# Urinary incontinence

## Data gathering

**History**  *Stress incontinence*: coughing, sneezing, laughing
*Urge incontinence*: frequency day and night, urge
*Obstructive incontinence*: hesitancy, poor stream/dribbling, nocturia, incomplete emptying
*Passive incontinence*: passing urine without realising
*Vaginal prolapse*: sensation of bearing down or lump vaginally
*UTI*: dysuria, fever
*Fluids*: evening, caffeine, alcohol
*GI symptoms*, e.g. constipation
*Past medical history*
   CVA, spinal problems, obstetrics, surgery
*Drug history*
   Diuretics, TCAs

**Red flags**  Haematuria
?Prostate cancer in men

**Examination**  Abdomen, *per vagina*, *per rectum*, external genitalia
Bladder, kidney
Enlarged prostate, constipation
Pelvic masses, vaginitis,?vaginal prolapse (use Sims speculum)
Inguinal herniae

## Interpersonal skills

**ICE**  Effect on life and self esteem, embarrassment
**For patient**  *"Stress incontinence is usually due to weak muscles in pelvic floor and occurs when coughing, sneezing or laughing due to increased pressure on bladder at these times"*
*"Urge incontinence is due to an overactive bladder when the muscle wall of the bladder contracts when it is not meant to. This causes an urgent desire to pass urine"*

# Management

*Investigations*   Urine dip and MCS
U&Es, glucose
Urinary diary

*Management*   Support
District nurse – incontinence pads, catheters
*Stress incontinence*
  Stop smoking, alcohol and caffeine
  Weight loss, avoid constipation
  Pelvic floor exercises for 3 months +/– physiotherapy
  Prolapse: ring pessary, surgery
*Urge incontinence*
  Bladder retraining – less frequent urination
  Oxybutinin 2.5–5 mg bd
  Tolterodine 1–2 mg bd

*Safety net*   Refer if:
- not responding to treatment
- unsure of diagnosis
- significant prolapse
- surgery is needed – urodynamic studies
- ?prostate cancer/red flags

# Testicular pain

## Data gathering

**History**    Trauma
Recent illness (mumps), fever
GU symptoms: irritative (frequency, urgency, dysuria), urethral discharge
GI symptoms: abdominal pain, vomiting, bowel habit
Sexual history if ?STI-related

**Red flags**    Cancer: weight loss, anorexia, lethargy
Torsion
Testicular lump

**Examination**    Abdomen, penis/scrotum +/– transillumination

## Interpersonal skills

**ICE**    Chaperone

## Management

**Investigations**    Testicular ultrasound
Urine dipstick and MCS
STI screen

**Management**    Analgesia, wait and see
Regular testicular self-examination
Epididymitis: urethral swab (gonorrhoea, chlamydia), Rx doxycycline and
either oral cefixine or IM ceftriazone +/– GU clinic referral

**Safety net**    Refer immediately if very painful/torsion
Refer using 2 week rule if ?cancer

Consider differential diagnosis: renal colic, hernia, groin strain.

# Lower urinary tract symptoms (LUTS) in men

*Summary of NICE Guidelines (2010)*

### Refer if any of following:
- not responding to conservative or drug treatment
- recurrent/persistent UTIs
- urinary retention
- renal impairment that could be due to lower urinary tract pathology
- suspected cancer
- stress incontinence

### General management
- For storage LUTS (especially incontinence) offer pads/collecting device until formal diagnosis made.
- "Active surveillance" is an option for mild–moderate symptoms (i.e. treat conservatively and monitor regularly).
- Bladder training is advised for storage symptoms/overactive bladder.
- Surgery is more effective for proven outflow tract obstruction compared to bladder training.

### Choice of drug
Offer medication only if conservative measures failed/inappropriate:
- *alpha blocker* (-osin) should be offered for moderate to severe LUTS
- *anticholinergics* offered for symptoms of overactive bladder (storage symptoms)
- *5-alpha reductase inhibitor* for LUTS and large prostate (>30 g)
- late afternoon *loop diuretic** for nocturia
- *oral desmopressin** for nocturia if medical causes excluded; need to measure serum sodium 3 days after first dose (stop if low)

*Currently unlicensed uses.

### Drug combinations
- Use alpha blocker with 5-alpha reductase inhibitor if more severe symptoms or PSA >1.4 ng/ml.
- Can use anticholinergic with alpha blocker if storage symptoms persist after alpha blocker alone.

### *Do not routinely offer:*

- cystoscopy
- imaging upper urinary tract
- flow-rate/post-void residual measurements
- penile clamps

# Chlamydia

*Based on BASHH (2006) and SIGN (2010) Guidelines*

## Data gathering

| | |
|---|---|
| *Symptoms* | Women: vaginal discharge, IMB/PCB, deep dyspareunia, lower abdominal pain<br>Men: urethral discharge, dysuria, epididymo-orchitis<br>Both: urethritis, reactive arthritis |
| *Sexual history* | Establish risk of other STIs<br>Sexually active, type of sex, sex with men/women<br>Contraception: condoms, IUS/IUD<br>Partners, previous partners, partner's sexual history<br>Previous STIs |
| *Social history* | Of patient and partner:<br>• travel<br>• IVDU |
| *Red flags* | PID: fever, acute pain, malaise<br>Rectal infection<br>Indicators of child sexual abuse |
| *Examination* | Women: PID, inflamed cervix +/– contact bleeding<br>Men: epididymo-orchitis |

## Interpersonal skills

| | |
|---|---|
| *ICE* | Respect patient's confidentiality<br>Non-judgemental<br>Clearly explain potential complications<br>*"Do you mind if I ask a few more personal questions?"* |
| *For patient* | *"Often has no symptoms"*<br>*"Condoms are the only effective means of preventing STIs (apart from abstinence)"*<br>Importance of complying with treatment (to avoid transmission and complications) and contact tracing<br>Avoid all sex (oral/vaginal/anal, even with condom) until treatment completed for both patient and partner (7 days after stat azithromycin) |

# Management

*Investigations*  Women: endocervical swab, low vulval self-swab or first void urine
Men: first void urine for chlamydia and gonorrhoea
*Other STIs*
Encourage screening for gonorrhoea, HIV, hepatitis B and syphilis

*Management*  *Conservative*
Testing for other STIs, preferably before treatment given
Contact tracing (via patient or provider)
Barrier contraception: condoms
*Medical*
Antibiotics (warn regarding interaction with COCP)
E.g. azithromycin* 1 g stat, or doxycycline 100 mg bd for 7 days

*Safety net*  *Review all infected patient in 2–4 weeks*
Contact tracing
Refer PID and rectal chlamydia to GUM clinic

*Available over the counter as Clamelle.

# Offer screening

- Annual screening for all sexually active people younger than 25 years of age (= *National Screening Programme*).
- If new sexual partner, or >1 sexual partner in the past 12 months.
- All men and women with another sexually transmitted infection, including genital warts.
- Sexual partners of those with proven or suspected chlamydial infection.
- Parents of infants with chlamydial conjunctivitis or pneumonitis.
- Semen and egg donors.
- Those who request screening.

**Offer screening to women:**
- before TOP
- before undergoing cervical instrumentation (e.g. IUD fitting)

# Chlamydia testing

*Women*:
- symptomatic: endocervical swab = best (remove excess cervical secretions first)
- asymptomatic: low vulval self-swab or first void urine

*Men*: first void urine = best; also urethral swab

*Men who have sex with men/anal sex*: also do rectal swabs

## Test for cure

- No routine need to re-test to check cure.
- If pregnant, should test for cure routinely.

## Complications

- Subfertility/infertility, possibly in men as well as women.
- Ectopic pregnancy.
- PID.

# Chronic kidney disease

*Based on Renal Association, NICE and SIGN Guidelines (2008)*

## Data gathering

| | |
|---|---|
| *History* | Fatigue, malaise |
| | *GI*: anorexia, nausea, vomiting |
| | *GU*: nocturia, polyuria |
| | *CCF*: SOB, ankle swelling |
| | *Past medical history/family history* |
| | Hypertension, CVD, DM, UTI, connective tissue diseases, cancer |
| | Renal disease |
| | *Drug history* |
| | NSAIDs, ACE inhibitors, diuretics, lithium |
| *Social history* | Smoking, alcohol |
| | Support |
| *Red flags* | Rapid deterioration in renal function (acute renal failure) |
| | Newly diagnosed renal dysfunction (assume this is acute renal failure until proven otherwise) |
| | Nephrotic syndrome |
| | Malignant hypertension |
| | Hyperkalaemia |
| *Examination* | BP, weight, fever |
| | Anaemia, uraemia |
| | CCF |
| | Palpable bladder |
| | Signs of underlying cause |

## Interpersonal skills

| | |
|---|---|
| *ICE* | Effect on life |

## Management

| | |
|---|---|
| *Investigations* | Urine dipstick (blood, protein) |
| | Urine MCS for ACR and casts |
| | FBC, U&Es, estimated GFR, LFTs, cholesterol, calcium, phosphate, bicarbonate, glucose |

Hepatitis screen, rheumatology screen, HIV
USS renal tract
(also CT/MRI, renal biopsy in secondary care)

**Management**  *Conservative*
Smoking cessation, weight loss, exercise
Low salt and low alcohol diet
*Medical*
Tight control of blood pressure (SBP <130)
Avoid NSAIDs and nephrotoxic drugs
ACE inhibitor if microalbuminuria (monitor U&Es and potassium)

**Safety net**  Monitor U&Es, CVD risk (BP, cholesterol)
Urgent referral if red flags

# Management of CKD in primary care

*Based on Renal Association, NICE and SIGN Guidelines*

| CKD stage | GFR (ml/ min) | Test frequency | Management |
|---|---|---|---|
| I | >90 | 12 monthly | Normal if no other evidence of kidney damage* |
| II | 60–90 | 12 monthly | Normal if no other evidence of kidney damage* |
| III | 30–60 | 6–12 monthly | Routinely refer if:<br>• progressively worsening renal functioning<br>• anaemia<br>• electrolyte imbalance<br>• microscopic haematuria or elevated protein: creatinine ratio<br>• uncontrolled BP<br>• systemic illness suspected, e.g. SLE<br>Check parathyroid hormone at diagnosis (if raised check vitamin D levels, refer if still raised despite adequate vitamin D replacement)<br>Immunisation: influenza, pneumococcus |
| IV | 15–30 | 3–6 monthly | Urgent referral (routine if known stable CKD IV)<br>3-monthly U&Es, FBC, calcium, phosphate, bicarbonate, parathyroid hormone<br>Immunisation: hepatitis B |
| V | <15 | 3 monthly | Immediate referral |

*Patients with no evidence of kidney damage and GFR >60 ml/min are assumed not to have CKD.

## Evidence of chronic kidney damage

- Persistent microalbuminuria, proteinuria, haematuria (exclude urological causes).
- Structural abnormalities of the kidney.
- Glomerulonephritis on biopsy.

## Proteinuria

- Exclude UTI.
- Confirm with early morning urine sample sent to laboratory (to exclude postural proteinuria).

- Persistent proteinuria – at least 2 tests, 1–2 weeks apart.
- Refer to nephrology if:
  - urine ACR >70
  - reduced GFR

# Haematuria

- Exclude infection, trauma and menstruation.
- No need for laboratory confirmation.
- Check U&Es and for proteinuria.
- All persistent haematuria requires further investigation (see **Haematuria** case).

# Refer for investigation for renal artery stenosis

- BP >150/90 despite three anti-hypertensive agents.
- Recurrent pulmonary oedema despite normal echo.
- Rising serum creatinine with raised CVD risk.
- Unexplained hypokalaemia with hypertension.

# Menorrhagia

*Based on NICE Guidelines (2007)*

## Data gathering

*History*    How much blood?
- number of towels, soaked through, flooding
- clots
- days of bleeding

When did heavy periods start?

Sudden change?

*Associated symptoms*
Painful periods, pelvic pain/pressure
Thyroid disturbance

*Anaemia*
SOB, fatigue

*Gynaecology history*
Periods – regular, IMB, PCB, LMP
Smear
Sexual activity + STI risk/discharge
Contraception

*Obstetric history*

*Past medical history/family history*
Bleeding disorders

*Drug history*
Aspirin, anticoagulants

*Social history*

*Red flags*    >45 years, sudden onset
Organic cause: IMB, PCB, pelvic mass, PID

*Examination*    Chaperone, permission
Consider pelvic examination if suspecting structural abnormality

## Interpersonal skills

*ICE*    Treatments already tried, effect on life

*For patient*    *"Heavy periods are common"*
*"Often no cause can be found"*
*"Usually responds to medication"* (note that IUS is NICE first-line)
*"Medications and Mirena IUS do not affect future fertility"*

# Management

| | |
|---|---|
| *Investigations* | All women should have FBC |
| | TFTs if symptomatic |
| | Coagulation screen if since menarche +/– family history |
| | FSH if menopausal |
| | STI screen if at risk of infection |
| | Ultrasound scan if there is a possibility of a structural abnormality |

*Management*

*Conservative*
    Menstrual diary

*Medical*
    Tranexamic acid: 1–1.5 g tds–qds at start of heavy bleeding for 5 days
    Mefanamic acid: 250–500 mg tds (better for pain)
    COCP
    Progestogens:
    • oral, e.g. norethisterone
    • injectable, e.g. depo-provera

*Surgical*
    Mirena IUS (NICE first-line), especially if contraception needed
    Transcervical resection of endometrium, endometrial laser ablation,
        hysterectomy

*Safety net*    Refer if red flags or ineffective treatment

# Amenorrhoea/oligomenorrhoea

## Data gathering

*History*   *Primary*
  "Have you ever had periods?"
  Menarche
  Genetic factors/family history
*Secondary (usually hormonal)*
  *Weight loss:*
    Stress/depression/eating disorders/exercise
  *Pregnancy:*
    "Is there a possibility you could be pregnant?"
    LMP, sexual activity, wanting to become pregnant?
  *Hyperprolactinaemia:*
    Galactorrhoea, bitemporal hemianopia
  *PCOS:*
    Hirsutism, acne, weight gain
  *Menopause:*
    Hot flushes, mood change, concentration, vaginal dryness
  *Hypo/hyperthyroidism/Cushing's:*
    Lethargy, skin changes
*Drug history*
    COCP, steroids, antipsychotics, chemo/radiotherapy

*Social history*

*Red flags*   Pelvic mass
  Signs of prolactinoma: galactorrhoea, bitemporal hemianopia

*Examination*   Secondary sexual characteristics
  BP, weight
  Cranial nerves if prolactinoma is suspected
  *Gynae*: smear, bimanual, speculum
  Pelvic ultrasound scan rather than examination if young girl

## Interpersonal skills

*ICE*   Chaperone
  Effect on life

# Management

*Investigations*   Rule out pregnancy
FSH/LH, testosterone, prolactin, SBHG
TFTs, glucose
Pelvic ultrasound scan

*Management*   If normal – reassurance
If patient wanting to get pregnant – refer for ?clomiphene

*Safety net*   Refer as per cause

- Primary amenorrhoea = no periods by 16 years of age, refer to gynaecology.
- Beware girl who has recently stopped COCP – wait 3–6 months.

# Premenstrual syndrome

## Data gathering

*History*  Bloating, breast pain, irritability and mood swings, reduced libido
Effect on life
Periods, bleeding, smear, contraception, obstetric history

*Social history*  Smoking, alcohol

*Red flags*

*Examination*

## Interpersonal skills

*ICE*  Depression, anxiety, stressors, effect on life
Initial open questions are important to identify symptoms:
*"No specific test for premenstrual symptoms, diagnosed on symptoms and their timing"*
*"Exact cause is unknown but lifestyle and hormonal factors are thought to play a role"*

## Management

*Investigations*

*Management*  Support, reassurance
3 months menstrual diary
*Conservative*
Exercise – menstrual diary
Diet
Stop smoking, healthy lifestyle, alcohol
Relaxation
*Medical*
Evening primrose oil
Vitamin B6 from day 14 to menses
Calcium supplements for breast tenderness, headaches, cramps
NSAIDs
COCP
Luteal progesterone
SSRIs

*Safety net*

# Polycystic ovary syndrome

## Data gathering

| | |
|---|---|
| *Presentation* | Weight gain |
| | Acne |
| | Difficulty in conceiving |
| *History* | "*Any unusual hair growth?*" |
| | Periods, oligomenorrhoea, LMP |
| | "*Are you trying to become pregnant?*" |
| | Obs and gynae history |
| *Social history* | Smoking |
| *Red flags* | |
| *Examination* | BP, weight |
| | Acne, hirsutism |

## Interpersonal skills

| | |
|---|---|
| *ICE* | Fertility, appearance/self esteem |
| *For patient* | "*Cause is unknown*" |
| | "*Common: 1 in 10–20 women have varying degrees of this*" |
| | "*Lifestyle changes are an important component of managing this condition*" |
| | "*Cysts develop within ovaries*" |
| | "*Ovaries do not regularly release eggs which can make it more difficult to become pregnant*" |
| | "*High levels of male hormones (androgens) can cause excessive hair growth*" |

## Management

| | |
|---|---|
| *Investigations* | Raised LH and testosterone |
| | Low SHBG |
| | Glucose, cholesterol, TFTs |
| | Ultrasound scan for polycystic ovaries |
| *Management* | *Conservative* |
| | Reassure that it is a common condition |
| | Weight loss, diet, exercise |

    Smoking cessation
    Contraception
*Medical*
    COCP if not wanting pregnancy
    Co-cyprindiol (Dianette) for acne, hirsutism and contraception
    Metformin – helps ovulation, oligomenorrhoea
*Fertility*: clomiphene – if wanting child (refer to gynaecology, high success rates)
Treat hirsutism and acne

### Safety net

[**Note**] Caution in prescribing COCP if raised BMI >30.

# Hirsutism

## Data gathering

**History**   Recent onset vs. longstanding
*PCOS*
   Periods, acne, weight gain, subfertility
*Family history*
   Ethnic origin
*Drug history*
   Phenytoin, steroids, ciclosporin

**Red flags**   Galactorrhoea
Recent onset and rapidly worsening
Pelvic mass
Virilisation

**Examination**   Weight, BMI, BP
Hair pattern, acne
Bimanual vaginal examination – if suspect ovarian/androgen secreting
   tumour

## Interpersonal skills

**ICE**   Effect on life and self-esteem
*"There is no cure but there are treatments to manage the condition"*

## Management

**Investigations**   Not needed if longstanding and regular periods
Testosterone, LH, FSH

**Management**   *Conservative*
   Support
   Weight loss if overweight
*Cosmetic*
   Bleaching, shaving, waxing, hair-removal creams, electrolysis
*Medical*
   Dianette – establish risk of CVD and DVT/PE first (smoking, weight, family
     history, etc.)
   Spironolactone
   Eflornithine cream (Vaniqa) – only if other drugs not working

***Safety net***    Refer if red flags or resistant to treatment

Think: could this be PCOS or "metabolic syndrome"?

- Hirsutism = *male-pattern* excess hair.
- Affects 1 in 10 women.
- Most is familial.
- Distinguish recent vs. longstanding.

# Combined oral contraceptive pill

Stopping ovulation is the main mechanism of action; it also thickens cervical mucus and causes endometrial changes.

Over 99% effective when taken properly.

See UKMEC criteria for more details on cautions and contraindications to using COCP.

| Disadvantages | Advantages |
|---|---|
| 1.2 x relative risk of breast cancer | 50% reduction in ovarian + uterine cancer |
| DVT (15–30/100 000 compared to 5/100 000 background or 60/100 000 pregnant) | |
| 5% develop hypertension after 5 years Smoking gives 3-times increased risk of vascular disease | No known increased MI risk |

| Absolute CI | Relative CI (don't give if more than one present) |
|---|---|
| DVT Heart disease Hypercholesterolaemia Focal migraine with aura Cancer of breast/cervix Sickle cell disease Smoking >40 cigarettes a day BMI >39 BP >160/95 Age >50 years | Family history of arterial disease or VTE Hypertension Smoking Obesity Age >35 years Migraine without aura |

## Side effects

Breakthrough bleeding – settles by 3 months.

Nausea, breast tenderness, bloating, PMT, mood change, vaginal discharge.

## Examination

Weight, BP, smear status.

## Management

Start day 1–5 of menstrual cycle, no extra precautions needed.

If started at any other time, need to use extra protection for 7 days (e.g. condoms or abstinence).

## Follow up

At 3 months, then 6–12 months.

Check smoking, BP, weight, smear status, new risk factors.

## Breakthrough bleeding

*Causes:* STI, enzyme inducers, pregnancy, compliance/vomiting, cervical lesions.

*Management:*
- investigate after 3 months – examine, swabs, consider ultrasound scan
- try pill with different progesterone or higher oestrogen

## No withdrawal bleed

Consider pregnancy, change to lower progesterone COCP.

## Stopping pill to conceive

Ideally use condoms for 3 months until normal period passed.

# Emergency contraception

## Data gathering

*History*   *"Why do you need the morning after pill?"*
When had unprotected sex? Any other times had sex? With whom?
Consensual sex?
*Contraception*
What do you normally use for contraception?
Why failed? How many missed pills?
*Contraindications*
History of pelvic infections
Ectopic pregnancies
*Past medical history*
Valvular heart disease
*Drug history*
*STI risk*
Regular partner?

*Social history*   STI risk

*Red flags*   STI, ?pregnant/LMP
Rape or vulnerable adult

*Examination*   BP, weight

## Interpersonal skills

*ICE*   *"How important is it that you do not become pregnant?"*

## Management

*Investigations*

*Management*   *"No contraceptive is 100% effective"*
Morning after pill
Copper IUD

*Safety net*   *"You should have a pregnancy test if your next period is abnormally light or delayed"*
*"Return promptly if any lower abdominal pain"*
*"Barrier contraception needed until next period"*
Long term contraception

STI risk/screen
Smears up to date
Vulnerability

# Levonorgestrel 1.5 mg single dose (Levonelle)

- Licensed up to 72 hours. Should be taken as soon as possible after UPSI.
- Inform patient *"effectiveness rapidly decreases with delay in using it"*.
- If vomit within 2 hours, take another dose (<1 in 20 women).
- May have some light bleeding or spotting.
- Can be taken more than once within a menstrual cycle.

# Ulipristal 30 mg single dose (EllaOne)

- Licensed up to 120 hours (5 days). Should be taken as soon as possible after UPSI.
- Inform patient *"effectiveness rapidly decreases with delay in using it"*.
- If vomit within 3 hours, take another dose (<1 in 20 women).
- Need to use barrier contraception or abstain until next period.
- Cannot use twice within the same menstrual cycle.

# Copper-containing IUD = most effective method

- *"Small device which contains copper put into your womb"*.
- Effective up to 5 days, or 5 days after ovulation.
- Take swabs.
- Antibiotic cover.

*Contraindications:*
- Pregnancy, severe anaemia, immunosuppression.
- Recent STI, PID.
- Unexplained PV bleeding.
- Genital malignancy.
- Copper – copper allergy, Wilson's.

# Termination of pregnancy request

## Data gathering

| | |
|---|---|
| *History* | *"How did you find out you were pregnant?"* |
| | Were you using contraception at the time? (split condom/missed pill) |
| | With regular partner? |
| | Does he know you are pregnant? |
| | Was sex consensual? |
| | *Social context* |
| |    Why do you want an abortion? |
| |    Have you spoken to anyone else about this? |
| | *Date pregnancy* |
| |    LMP? Normal period? |
| | *Past medical history* |
| |    Gynae/obs, psychiatric history |
| *Social history* | Home, work, children, relationships |
| *Red flags* | Socially isolated, domestic violence, abuse |
| | Lower abdominal pain |
| *Examination* | BP, BMI |

## Interpersonal skills

| | |
|---|---|
| *ICE* | Ensure patient makes best decision for her and is well supported |
| | Note that the patient's partner cannot give consent for or refuse a TOP. |

## Management

| | |
|---|---|
| *Investigations* | Pregnancy test |
| *Management* | *"Are you aware of your options?"* |
| | *"How sure are you that you want an abortion?"* |
| | Obliged to go though some options with patient before proceeding: |
| |   &bull; have baby |
| |   &bull; adoption |
| |   &bull; TOP – medical/surgical |
| | Refer for TOP, e.g. to local Marie Stopes Clinic |
| *Safety net* | Long term contraception/STI screen |
| | Psychological and emotional support |

# 1967 Abortion Act

Allows TOP at any stage in pregnancy in NHS hospital if:
- risk to life of mother
- risk of grave permanent injury to the mother's physical/mental health
- substantial risk that child would be seriously handicapped.

Allows TOP before 24 weeks gestation if:
- reduces the risk to a woman's life
- reduces the risk to her physical or mental health
- reduces the risk to physical or mental health of her existing children
- the baby is at substantial risk of being seriously mentally or physically handicapped.

# Complications of termination

- Infection – 5%, minimised by antibiotics and pre-procedure screening.
- Cervical trauma – 1%, less risk in early termination.
- Rare: haemorrhage (1.5/1000), perforation of uterus (1–4/1000), failed termination (2–5/1000).
- No evidence to link termination with subsequent infertility or pre-term delivery.

# Psychological effects

- Only long term in small proportion.
- Early distress is common – usually a continuation of the symptoms present before abortion.
- Remember negative effects on both the mother and the child where abortion has been denied.

# At under 7 weeks' gestation

Medical abortion, e.g. Mifepristone orally followed after 48 h by Gemeprost vaginally. Avoid suction termination.

# At 7–15 weeks' gestation

- Conventional suction termination is appropriate. Local or general anaesthesia.
- Medical abortion may be preferable above 12 weeks.

# Terminations at >15 weeks' gestation

Dilatation and evacuation, preceded by preparation or medical abortion.

# Subfertility

## Data gathering

*History*  How long trying to conceive? Without contraception?
How often having sex? Any problems with sex?
Either partner had a child?
Previous pregnancies? Miscarriage? TOP?
Regular periods?
*Past medical history*
    General health, STI risk
    *Female*: surgery including appendectomy, rubella vaccination
    *Male*: testicular trauma, mumps, varicocoele
*Drug history*
    NSAIDs may impair fertility, antipsychotics, teratogens

*Social history*  Smoking, alcohol, recreational drugs
Stress

*Red flags*  STI, chronic disease, pelvic pathology, ambiguous genitalia

*Examination*  *Female*
    BMI, BP, hirsutism/androgenisation
    Abnormal genitalia, pelvic mass
*Male*
    Gynaecomastia, abnormal genitalia, inguinal hernia, testicles

## Interpersonal skills

*ICE*  Preferably joint consultation with both partners; important to investigate
    both partners
Difficult to cover all in single consultation, may need to schedule another
    consultation
*"Do you have any idea why you are having difficulties becoming pregnant?"*

*For patient*  *"Subfertility affects 1 in 6 couples"*

## Management

*Investigations*  *Female*
        STI screen
        LH, FSH, luteal progesterone, prolactin, TFTs
        Transvaginal ultrasound

*Male*
> Semen analysis

***Management***   Reassurance: *"over 80% of healthy couples having regular sex (2–3 times per week, without contraception) conceive within 12 months"*
*Conservative*
> Pre-conception advice – folic acid, smoking cessation, alcohol, weight, diet, etc.
> Sexual intercourse 2–3 times a week

*Medical*
> Clomiphene

*Surgical*
> *In-vitro* fertilisation, intracytoplasmic sperm injection

***Safety net***   Refer as per local criteria to assisted conception unit or equivalent, e.g. typically:
- no conception after 18 months
- woman between 35 and 40 years of age with no living child

Abnormal investigations – refer as per cause

# Screening

## Cervical screening

To *prevent* cancer (not cure it; detects pre-cancerous lesions):
- 25–64 years of age: 3-yearly for 25–49 year-olds, 5-yearly for 50–64 year-olds
- >65 years if previous abnormal smear or no smear since 50 years

2000 new cases cervical cancer/year, most of these women have not had recent smear.
- 1 in 20 are borderline, very few develop cancer
- 1 in 20 are mild dyskaryosis, cancer very unlikely
- 1 in 100 are moderate dyskaryosis, pre-cancerous, intermediate probability of developing cancer

Risk factors for cervical cancer include smoking, HPV infection, COCP.

| Screening result | Action |
|---|---|
| Negative | Inform patient, routine recall |
| Inadequate | Repeat as soon as possible (definitely within 3 months) Refer colposcopy if three consecutive inadequate smears |
| Borderline | Endocervical cells: refer colposcopy Squamous cells: <ul><li>repeat within 6 months</li><li>three consecutive negatives 6 months apart before routine recall</li></ul> |
| Mild dyskaryosis | Ideally refer colposcopy Can repeat in 6 months – if negative, need three negatives 6 months apart before routine recall |
| Moderate/severe dyskaryosis | Refer colposcopy |

## Colposcopy

"A more detailed examination of the cervix."
- The doctor uses a speculum and magnifier (colposcope).
- A liquid is used to "paint" the cervix which shows up the abnormal cells.
- Takes 10–15 mins.
- Biopsy often taken.

Treatments can be undertaken – cryotherapy, laser treatment, loop diathermy.
- Few weeks for the cervix to heal after treatment.
- Once it has healed, a normal sex life can be resumed.
- Does not affect fertility.

## Breast cancer screening

50–70 year olds, 3 yearly mammograms (available to patients >65 years on request).

# Diagnosing menopause

Defined as no periods for 2 years in those patients <50 years or 1 year for patients >50 years.

## Data gathering

*History* Bleeding pattern, LMP
*Symptoms*
　Flushes/sweats
　Vaginal dryness, urinary incontinence
　Anxiety, depression
*Gynae history*
　Smears, mammograms, contraception

*Social history* Smoking, alcohol

*Red flags* Abnormal bleeding: irregular, painful, PCB, bleeding 1 year after LMP

*Examination* BP, weight, breasts

## Interpersonal skills

*ICE* Depression, anxiety, effect on life

*For patient* *"This is when the ovaries stop producing as much oestrogen (female hormone). This causes your periods to gradually stop"*

## Management

*Investigations* Consider pregnancy test and TFTs
FSH if uncertain of diagnosis: e.g. <45 years, hysterectomy, on HRT/COCP/POP/IUS

*Management* Check patient's understanding
Stressors
Discuss HRT
Lifestyle: exercise and diet (healthy diet and avoid spicy foods)
Flushes and sweats: deep breathing exercises, cool environment, loose clothing, evening primrose oil
Topical oestrogens: help vaginal dryness and reduce UTIs.

*Safety net* Should investigate:
- irregular or painful bleeding/PCB
- bleeding 1 year after LMP

# Starting hormone replacement therapy

*Why start?*   Control menopausal symptoms
Osteoporosis prevention if <50 years (e.g. hysterectomised)

*Risk factors*   Smoking
Past medical history or family history of breast cancer and PE/DVT
Mammograms not up to date

*Contraindications*  Breast or endometrial cancer
DVT/PE
Severe liver/kidney/gallbladder disease
Otosclerosis (may worsen on HRT)

*Side effects*   Spotting for first 3 months
Fluid retention, breast enlargement

| Advantages | Disadvantages |
|---|---|
| Controls symptoms<br>Prevents osteoporosis and colon cancer<br>Decreases UTIs | Small increase in breast cancer, PE/DVT and stroke<br>  &bull; 6/1000 extra cases breast cancer after 5 years<br>  &bull; excess risk disappears 5 years after stopping<br>  &bull; no increased risk of breast cancer if <50 years |

| Cyclical combined | Non-cyclical combined (continuous) |
|---|---|
| Normally start with cyclical preparations<br>Start on 1st 5 days of cycle<br>For women with periods<br>Perimenopausal women<br>Women will continue to have regular periods on this preparation | Women without periods (for at least 1 year)<br>Hysterectomised<br>Been on cyclical for several years and wish to stop periods<br>Tibolone is non-cyclical, less breast cancer risk<br>Women will not have periods on this preparation |

- Women without uterus can have oestrogen alone (less risk of breast cancer).
- Tibolone: for women who cannot take oestrogens, protects against osteoporosis, helps symptoms.

- SSRIs can be effective in women where HRT in contraindicated.
- Do not use topical oestrogens for more than 1 year at a time.
- Can give HRT as patch, implant or orally.
- Can give low dose COCP in fit non-smokers to relieve symptoms of menopause.
- HRT is <u>not</u> contraception.

## Follow up

- Every 3 months initially, then every 6–12 months.
- Ask about abnormal bleeding.
- Some women have no bleeds on continuous preps – this can be normal, exclude pregnancy.
- Most women only need up to 5 years of HRT.
- Examination: BP, weight, smears, mammograms.

# Antenatal counselling

*Based on NICE Guidelines (2008)*

Assessment of gestational age should be based on an early ultrasound scan rather than the last menstrual period.

| | |
|---|---|
| *Folic acid* | 400 µg of folic acid up to 12 weeks to reduce neural tube defects<br>5 mg if high risk suggested by past medical history or family history (coeliac, DM, sickle cell disease, anticonvulsants) |
| *Vitamin D* | 10 µg per day during pregnancy and breastfeeding<br>High risk groups:<br>• darker skin colour<br>• reduced sunlight exposure (e.g. housebound, remain covered when outdoors)<br>• diet lacking eggs/oily fish/meat<br>• BMI >30 |
| *Rubella* | Immunisation if needed |
| *Nutrition* | Normal diet, five portions of fruit and vegetables per day<br>Drinking plenty of milk to raise stores of vitamins, iron and calcium is reasonable<br>Avoid:<br>• uncooked meat, fish and eggs (toxoplasmosis)<br>• liver (vitamin A)<br>• milk that has not been pasteurised<br>• soft cheeses (listeria)<br>• all fruit and vegetables should be washed (toxoplasmosis)<br>• herbal preparations, caffeine |
| *Exercise* | Gentle programme of regular exercise if not already<br>Avoid high impact/contact sports, especially if risk of falls or abdominal trauma<br>Avoid excessive heating, hot tubs/saunas, scuba diving (birth defects, decompression) |
| *Drug history* | As few medicines as possible, including OTC medications |
| *Smoking* | Avoid smoking, including cannabis<br>NRT safer than smoking (lower dose nicotine, be sure to take patches off at night)<br>(Zyban/Champix are contraindicated in pregnancy) |

| | |
|---|---|
| *Alcohol* | Avoid (1–2 drinks twice a week unlikely to be harmful) |
| | Avoid binge drinking and intoxication |
| *Social history* | Maternity rights and benefits |
| | Reassure patient it is safe to continue working |
| | Check occupation for exposure to harmful agents |

[**Note**] Do not recommend routine iron supplementation.

# Common issues during pregnancy

### Nausea and vomiting during pregnancy

- Generally resolves by 14–16 weeks of gestation.
- Frequent and small meals.
- Avoid greasy/spicy foods.
- Antihistamines = first-line medical treatment (e.g. promethazine).
- Ginger and P6 acupressure may be beneficial.
- Red flags: dehydration.
- Think: could this be UTI or hydatidiform mole?

### Heartburn during pregnancy

- Small regular meals.
- Avoid meals late at night.
- Raising the head of bed.
- Antacids.

### Travel

- ? Increased risk of DVT if flying.
- Compression hosiery.
- Also discuss vaccinations and travel insurance if travelling abroad.
- Car seat belts above and below bump rather than over it.
- Guidelines with air travel vary from airline to airline, but most will not allow women to travel if:
  - >36 weeks pregnant (>32 weeks if multiple pregnancies); airlines may require a certificate after 28 weeks stating the pregnancy is progressing normally
  - history of premature delivery
  - cervical incompetence
  - PV bleeding

# Summary of NICE Guidelines (2008) on antenatal screening

### Haematological conditions

- Ideally before 10 weeks.
- Sickle-cell disease.
- Thalassaemia.

### Gestational diabetes

Screen high risk groups (if any of following risk factors present):

- BMI >30
- previous GDM or FH diabetes
- previous macrosomic baby >4.5 kg
- South Asian, Black Caribbean, Middle Eastern

### Down syndrome

- 1 in 1000 births; maternal age 30 years 1 in 500, 35 years 1 in 250, 40 years 1 in 60.
- Offer the "combined test" at 11–13 weeks (Nuchal scan, hCG, pregnancy-associated plasma protein A)

*Other options include:*

- chorionic villus sampling: 8–12 weeks, allows 1st trimester TOP, 1–2% miscarriage rate
- amniocentesis: at 15–16 weeks, TOP before 20 weeks, alpha fetoprotein takes 1 week, karyotype 3 weeks, 1% miscarriage rate

# Booking visit

*Based on NICE Guidelines (2008)*

## Data gathering

|                    |                                                                        |
|--------------------|------------------------------------------------------------------------|
| *History*          | *"How do you know you are pregnant?"*                                   |
|                    | LMP + calculate expected due date                                      |
|                    | *Patient and partner*                                                  |
|                    | Age, occupation, race                                                  |
|                    | Past medical history                                                   |
|                    | Family history                                                         |
|                    | Obs and gynae history                                                  |
| *Social history*   | Alcohol, smoking                                                       |
|                    | Social support, finances, home/work                                   |
| *Red flags*        | Family history, complex past medical/obstetric history                 |
|                    | Psychiatric history                                                    |
|                    | Domestic violence                                                      |
|                    | Female genital mutilation                                              |
| *Examination*      | Weight, BP                                                             |
|                    | Heart, chest, abdomen, legs (varicose veins)                          |
|                    | No need for vaginal examination                                       |

## Interpersonal skills

|       |                   |
|-------|-------------------|
| *ICE* | Effect on life    |
|       | Depression screen |

## Management

|                   |                                                                              |
|-------------------|------------------------------------------------------------------------------|
| *Investigations*  | Urine: dip + MSU (proteinuria and bacteriuria)                               |
|                   | STI, e.g. chlamydia screening especially in under 25s                        |
|                   | Bloods: FBC, ABO/rhesus, Hep B, HIV, +/– rubella status, haemoglobinopathies, syphilis |
| *Management*      | *"Do you have any ideas of how you want to proceed from here?"*              |
|                   | *Care*: shared/community/hospital                                            |
|                   | *Diet*: e.g. folic acid                                                      |
|                   | *Screening*: e.g. ultrasound scan at 12 and 20 weeks                         |
|                   | *Benefits*: free prescription and dental care for pregnancy and 12 months after |

*Safety net*     Refer if complex case

# Women requiring additional care during pregnancy

- Cardiac conditions (including HTN).
- Kidney disease.
- Endocrine disease.
- Diabetes requiring insulin.
- Haematological disorders.
- Epilepsy.
- Severe asthma.
- HIV.
- Hepatitis B.
- Mental illness.
- Illicit use of drugs, e.g. heroin, cocaine, ecstasy.
- BMI >30 or BMI <18.
- Vulnerable women (e.g. teenagers, those lacking support).
- Those at risk of complications, e.g. smokers, aged >40 years.

# Subsequent antenatal visits

## Data gathering

*History*  General health, problems, gestational age

*Social history*

*Red flags*  Bleeding, pain, mood, support

*Examination*  BP + urine dip
Fundal height
Fetus:
- movements/heartbeat from 12 weeks
- presentation from 32 weeks

## Interpersonal skills

*ICE*  Effect on life

## Management

*Investigations*  Screening tests
ABO and haemoglobin at 28 and 32 weeks

# Paediatrics – general approach

## Data gathering

| | |
|---|---|
| *History* | Past medical history |
| |     Birth history |
| |     Immunisations |
| |     Developmental history |
| |     Feeding/diet |
| | Family history |
| | Drug history |
| *Social history* | Family and siblings |
| | School |
| *Red flags* | Developmental delay, poor growth/weight gain |
| | Child protection issues, abuse/neglect |
| *Examination* | Plot on centile charts: height, weight, head circumference |
| | Alert, responsiveness, hydration |

## Interpersonal skills

| | |
|---|---|
| *ICE* | Concerns, empathy, effect on parents |
| | Watch out for postnatal depression |

# ADHD

## Data gathering

*History*  Three main features for at least 6 months in two different situations
(e.g. school and home):
1. inattention
2. hyperactivity
3. impulsiveness

Above must be abnormal for child's age
Normal developmental milestones?

*Social history*  How is child getting along at school? Friends?
Relationships within family, interaction with siblings
Interests and activities

*Red flags*  Abnormal development
Child protection issues

*Examination*  Height, weight, behaviour and interaction

## Interpersonal skills

*ICE*  Ensure child meets ADHD criteria
Empathy

*For patient*  *"There is no simple test to confirm ADHD"*
*"A specialist can assess your child to confirm the diagnosis and recommend treatment"*

## Management

*Investigations*

*Management*  Support and involve entire family in management
Family therapy
Diet: avoid caffeine and sugary foods/drinks
Regular exercise
Ignore bad behaviour, reward good behaviour
Medications should be started by specialists only

*Safety net*  Refer for assessment if meets criteria for ADHD
Regular review and support to family

# Nocturnal enuresis

*Based on NICE Guidelines (2010)*

Nocturnal enuresis = night time bed-wetting in a child > 5 years old.

## Data gathering

**History**   *Primary vs. secondary*
    Has child ever been dry?
    Wet during day?
*Psychological*
    Toilet habit, e.g. avoids using toilets at school
    Frequency and pattern of bedwetting, e.g. related to school or weekends?
    Sleeping environment, e.g. share a bed?
*Gastro-intestinal symptoms*
    Bowel habit, assess for constipation
*Fluid intake and caffeine*
*Family history*
    Bed wetting
    Siblings
*"Have you tried anything to prevent this already?"*

**Social history**   Family and school

**Red flags**   Poor growth and development
Behavioural problems
Daytime wetting after 4 years of age
Polyuria, polydipsia, weight loss (?type 1 diabetes)
Dysuria
Neurological symptoms
Suspicions of child maltreatment

**Examination**   Growth
Abdomen
Spine – sacral dimple/naevus/hair
Ankle jerks

## Interpersonal skills

**ICE**   Often the parent/carer may have difficulties coping or they may be expressing anger
*"How has this affected you/your family?"*

*For patient*   *"Delay in maturation of control mechanisms"*
                *"Bedwetting is not the fault of the child"*
                *"Can also be due to infection, caffeinated drinks, constipation and*
                    *psychological reasons"*
                *"1 in 10 five year olds wet their beds"*
                *"Bedwetting is very common under the age of 5 years"*
                *"Alarms have high long-term success rate"*
                *"Desmopressin reduces the amount of urine made by the kidneys and is*
                    *good for rapid short-term results"*

# Management

*Investigations*   Urine dip and MCS if recent onset, daytime enuresis, ?infection, ?DM

*Management*   *Conservative*
                Avoid evening/caffeinated drinks
                Ensure normal toilet habit
                +/– nappies/starter pants (younger children), bed protection/waterproof
                    mattress cover
                Ensure child has easy access to toilet at night, e.g. leave bathroom
                    light on
                Parental/carer support
                *Reward child* (e.g. star chart) if:
                - drinks appropriate amount of fluid during day
                - goes to toilet before bed – can lift child to lavatory when parents go to
                  bed
                - engaging in management (e.g. taking medication, helping to change
                  sheets)
                - dry nights
                *Specific treatments*
                First-line = enuresis alarm – most respond by 2–3 months, stop after
                    14 dry nights
                Second-line = desmopressin po/sl (not intranasal) at night, e.g. social
                    occasions

*Safety net*   Support and follow up
                Refer daytime wetting over 4 years of age to urology for neuropathic bladder
                **Think**: could this be diabetes or a UTI?

# Principles of management

- Involve parent and child, and health visitor/school nurse.
- Reward wanted behaviour.

- Ignore wet nights, no punishment.
- Give a treat if seven consecutive dry nights.
- Avoid punitive measures.
- Offer support for parent/carer if appropriate.

[**Note**] Specific treatments can be considered at any age (previous guidance suggested only those children >7 years old required specific treatment).

An alarm may be considered inappropriate if:
- bedwetting is infrequent (<1–2 episodes per week)
- parents/carers are having difficulty coping with the bedwetting
- parents/carers are expressing negativity/blame to the child

Secondary nocturnal enuresis = dry for 6 months beforehand.

# Constipation in children

*Based on NICE Guidelines (2010)*

## Data gathering

**History**   Try to identify what is meant by constipation, e.g. fewer motions? straining at stool? hard stools?

*Stool*
> Frequency: fewer than three complete motions per week
> Form: often large and hard or rabbit dropping
> Overflow: may be passed without sensation

*During defecation*
> Pain, bleeding, straining

*Diet and growth*
> Is child thriving?

*Past history*
> Constipation, fissure

**Social history**   Look for a precipitating factor, e.g. moving house, toilet training, illness, starting nursery/school, major change in family

**Red flags**   Constipation since birth/first few weeks of life
Obstruction (abdominal distension and/or vomiting)
Failure to pass meconium in newborn
PR bleeding, "Ribbon stools"
Leg weakness
Delayed locomotor development

**Examination**   Abdomen
Anus (ensure no suspicion of NAI)
Spine/gluteals (ensure no naevi, pits, scoliosis)
Elicit lower limb reflexes if red flags present
NICE advises the following regarding PR examination:
- only perform if you are competent at spotting Hirschsprung's disease
- do not perform PR if >1 year old and red flag present
- ensure chaperone present

## Interpersonal skills

**ICE**   Effect on school, other siblings, meal times, family dynamics

**For parent/ carer**   Up to one-third of children will be affected at some point

# Management

*Investigations*  TFTs

*Management*  Reassure underlying causes excluded if no red flags on Hx or examination
Explain may take several months for condition to resolve
Diet alone is <u>not</u> recommended as first line treatment
Tailor treatment to child's age
*Conservative*
  Diet: adequate fluid intake, high fibre
  Daily exercise
  Scheduled toileting (to achieve regular bowel habit)
  Bowel diary (e.g. Bristol stool scale)
  Reward system
*Medical*
  Movicol = first-line
  Stimulant laxative = second-line
  Add lactulose or docusate if hard stools

*Safety net*  If red flags refer urgently and do not treat for constipation.
If faltering growth, treat for constipation and test for coeliac disease and
  hypothyroidism.
Ensure no NAI.
Refer unresponsive idiopathic constipation
Review after 1 week if treating for faecal impaction

## Laxatives

Should be stopped gradually.

Should be continued for several weeks once normal bowel habit regained.

If child is toilet training, laxatives should be continued until toilet training completed.

## Faecal impaction

Suggested by overflow diarrhoea and faecal mass rectally or abdominally.
Disimpaction regime may cause initial increased soiling and abdominal pain.
Any child undergoing disimpaction should be reviewed after 1 week.

- Movicol at higher disimpaction dose = first line.
- Add stimulant laxative if disimpaction not achieved after 2 weeks.
- Lactulose is alternative if movicol not tolerated.
- Sodium citrate enemas and rectal medication only used if all oral medications have failed.
- Phosphate enemas only to be used under specialist supervision in hospital.

# Diarrhoea and vomiting in child under five

*Based on NICE Guidelines (2009)*

## Data gathering

|  |  |
|---|---|
| *History* | Diarrhoea, vomiting – number of episodes, bleeding, mucus |
|  | Other infective symptoms |
|  | *Hydration* |
|  |     Breastfeeding |
|  |     Ability to tolerate oral fluids |
|  |     Wetting nappies/urine output |
| *Social history* | Unwell contacts |
|  | Recent travel |
|  | Ability of parents to cope |
|  | Social circumstances |
| *Red flags* | Shock, drowsiness |
|  | Dehydration, sunken eyes, reduced skin turgor |
|  | Blood in stool |
| *Examination* | Dehydration, capillary refill time, skin turgor, fontanelle |
|  | Shock: tachypnoea/cardia, hypotension |
|  | Pulse/HR |
|  | Abdomen |
|  | Signs of other infection |

## Interpersonal skills

|  |  |
|---|---|
| *ICE* | Ability of parents to cope |
| *For parent/ carer* | *"Hand washing with soap, warm running water and careful drying most important to prevent spread."* |
|  | *"Wash hands before touching food, after changing nappies/going to toilet"* |
|  | *"Diarrhoea usually lasts 5–7 days and stops within 2 weeks"* |
|  | *"Vomiting usually lasts 1–2 days and stops within 3 days"* |
|  | Avoid school/nursery whilst symptomatic and for 48 hours afterwards |
|  | Most children can be safely managed at home |

# Management

*Investigations*   Stool MCS/OCP

*Management*   Hygiene
        Handwashing
        Avoid sharing towels
    Rehydration
        Rehydration, continue breastfeeding
        Avoid fruit juices or fizzy drinks until diarrhoea has stopped
        Advise parents how to recognise dehydration
    Social
        Avoid school/nursery whilst symptomatic and for 48 hours afterwards
        No swimming in pools for 2 weeks after last episode of diarrhoea

*Safety net*   Refer urgently for IV rehydration if dehydrated, unable to tolerate oral fluids
    Notify public health authority if suspect outbreak of gastroenteritis
    Advise parents of how and when to seek help

No antidiarrhoeals, no routine antibiotics

## Dehydration:

- cool peripheries
- pale/mottled skin
- sunken eyes
- dry mucous membranes

## Stool investigations if:

- suspect septicaemia
- blood or mucus in stool
- child is immunocompromised
- also consider if recent travel, diarrhoea not improving at day 7, or uncertain diagnosis

## Rehydration:

- encourage breastfeeding/milk/fluid intake
- ORS solution if increased risk dehydration
- avoid fruit juice/carbonated drinks

## After rehydration:

- reintroduce child's normal diet – e.g. full strength milk or solid foods
- avoid fruit juices or fizzy drinks until diarrhoea has stopped

## Parents should seek help if:

- not drinking oral fluids
- dehydration develops
- symptoms do not resolve as expected

# Eczema in children

*Based on NICE Guidelines (2007)*

## Data gathering

| | |
|---|---|
| *History* | Duration, site, itch |
| | Precipitant: allergen, washing powders, travel, soaps, stress |
| | Impact on life, sleep and self-esteem |
| | Growth and development |
| | *Past medical history/family history* |
| | Atopy: hayfever, asthma |
| | *Drug history* |
| | Treatments already tried |
| *Social history* | Psychological or social problems in child/carer/parent |
| | Housing/environmental issues |
| | School |
| *Red flags* | Secondary infection |
| | Failure to thrive |
| | GI symptoms (consider food allergy) |
| | Psychological or social problems in child/carer/parent |
| *Examination* | Distribution: flexural, seborrhoeic |
| | Erythema, papules, vesicles, crusting, weeping, dry |
| | Lichenification, scarring, excoriation |
| | Cushingoid appearance |

## Interpersonal skills

| | |
|---|---|
| *ICE* | Empathy with parent's situation |
| | Effect on child's life |
| | Psychological or social problems in child/carer/parent |
| *For parent/ carer* | *"Sometimes called dermatitis, inflammation of skin, itchy skin condition"* |
| | *"Controlled and not cured"* |
| | *"Children usually grow out of it, but it can occasionally persist"* |

## Management

| | |
|---|---|
| *Investigations* | Skin patch testing if contact dermatitis and unknown allergen |

*Management*  Avoid allergens, perfumed products, detergents (e.g. gloves when washing up)
*Medical*
Soap substitute, avoid soaps
Unperfumed emollients for washing, bathing and moisturising
Topical steroids (use mild strength, e.g. 1% hydrocortisone, for face or young children)
*Severe*
Wet wrapping over steroids/emollients if severe
Phototherapy
Immunosuppression: oral steroids, tacrolimus
*Infection*
Topical: fusidic acid cream (short courses to avoid resistance)
Oral: flucloxacillin, acyclovir (for herpes; refer same day)
*Other*
Antihistamine for itch (not for routine use)

*Safety net*  Regular review with compliance assessment
Refer if unresponsive to treatment (especially facial), severe, suspicion of herpes infection, recurrent infection
Refer same day if herpes infection

## Summary of NICE Guideline (2007) on eczema in children

- Most children with mild symptoms will not require allergy testing.
- Exclusion diets are controversial and generally only used with dietician advice in children.
- Complementary therapies: no good evidence base, caution against use.
- Continue treatment of flare-ups for 48 hours after symptoms resolve.
- Consider trial 1/12 with antihistamines if severe or itch pronounced, not for routine use.

### Infections

Usually *Staphylococcus aureus*/*Streptococcus*:
- first-line = flucloxacillin
- second-line = erythromycin
- third-line = clarithromycin

Antiseptics (e.g. chlorhexidine) can be used as adjuncts in recurrent infections.

Usually no need to take swabs unless suspect resistance or atypical infection.

### Herpes infection

Suspect if:
- infection not resolving on antibiotics

- rapidly worsening/painful
- fever, lethargy, distress
- clustered blisters
- punched out erosions (1–3 mm)

Treat with oral acyclovir and refer for same day dermatology advice.

If skin around eyes involved, refer for same day dermatology and ophthalmology advice.

# When to suspect child maltreatment

*Summary of NICE Guidelines (2009)*

Consider = maltreatment is one possible cause.

Suspect = serious level of concern of maltreatment, but not proof.

### Risk factors

- Parental/carer drug or alcohol abuse.
- Parent/carer mental health problems.
- History of violence in family.
- History of child maltreatment.
- History of animal maltreatment.
- Vulnerable and unsupported parent/carers.
- Disability in child.

### Types of maltreatment

- Physical abuse.
- Sexual abuse.
- Emotional abuse.
- Neglect.
- Fabricated or induced illness.

## Physical features

### Consider if:

- poor explanation of unusual/serious injury
- hypothermia, unexplained cold injuries (e.g. swollen red hands or feet)
- unexplained oral injuries
- delayed presentation
- hypernatraemia

### Suspect if:

- bruises in shape of hand/stick/teeth/grip/implement
- unexplained petechiae
- bruises/petechiae on neck (strangulation) or wrists (ligature marks)
- human bite (not caused by young child)
- unexplained lacerations/abrasions
- unexplained burns/scalds
- scalds indicating forced immersion: buttocks, lower limbs, glove or stocking distribution, sharply delineated borders
- fractures – e.g. breaks of different ages, rib fractures in infants, long bone fractures in immobile child

***"Shaking baby" causes (especially <3 years of age):***

- intracranial injury
- retinal haemorrhages
- subdural haemorrhages
- subarachnoid haemorrhage
- hypoxic–ischaemic damage to brain (suffocation)
- spinal injury
- intra-abdominal or intrathoracic injury

***Suspect above especially if:***

- immobile child
- symmetrical or multiple
- on areas usually protected by clothing
- on non-bony parts of face/body such as eye/ear/sides of face/buttocks
- in shape of implement/cigarette/iron

# Sexual abuse

Sex with a child <13 years = unlawful.

Therefore any pregnancy in girl <13 years = maltreatment.

***Consider if:***

- unexplained recurrent dysuria, anal or genital symptoms
- gaping anus (without neurological explanation or severe constipation)
- foreign body in vagina/anus (may cause offensive discharge)
- hepatitis B in young person (without vertical transmission)
- STI or anogenital warts in young person (without vertical transmission)
- pregnancy in young person

***Suspect if:***

- recurrent anal/genital symptom with behavioural/emotional change
- unexplained genital/anal/perianal injury
- unexplained anal fissure (e.g. no constipation or Crohn's disease)
- STI in child <13 years (without vertical transmission)
- sexualised behaviour in pre-pubertal child

# Neglect

Neglect = risk to the child.

Neglect = persistent failure to meet child's needs (physical/psychological).

Likely to result in impairment of health or development.

May not be deliberate.

Difficult for parents to achieve balance of giving child freedom to learn vs. risks, but persistent failure on part of parents may be neglect.

*Consider if:*

- severe/persistent infestations (scabies, head lice)
- parents/carers not giving essential prescribed medications to child
- untreated tooth decay
- fail to attend health promotion (immunisations, screening, reviews)
- consistently inappropriate clothing, e.g. for weather or size
- failure to thrive
- inadequate carer/supervision
- animal bite
- near drowning event with lack of supervision

*Suspect if:*

- medical advice not sought when it should be
- persistently smelly/dirty child, especially ingrained dirt
- poor home environment (hygiene, food provision, unsafe)

Abandonment = maltreatment.

# Behavioural features

*Consider if:*

- fearful/withdrawn
- aggressive/oppositional
- habitual body rocking
- indiscriminate affection seeking, overfriendly to strangers, excessive clinginess
- excessive good behaviour to prevent parental disapproval
- children with excessive responsibilities that interfere with school, etc.
- dissociation
- recurrent nightmares
- DSH
- secondary or nocturnal enuresis
- encopresis
- exposure to domestic abuse
- parent not facilitating child's social development
- punishing a child for wetting (if involuntary)

*Suspect if:*

- steals, scavenges food
- precocious/inappropriate sexual behaviour

# Fabricated illness

- Unexplained poor response to treatment (fabricated illness)
- New symptoms start as old ones stop
- Symptoms only with carer
- Multiple specialist opinions sought and disputed by carer
- Limited school attendance

# Depression

*Based on NICE Guidelines (2009) and SIGN Guidelines (2010)*

## Data gathering

**History**  *Screening questions*
Over the past month have you:
- felt down, depressed or hopeless?
- had little interest or pleasure in doing things?

*Biological features*
Unintentional weight loss?
*"How has your appetite been?"*
*"Are you sleeping well?"*

*Functional impairment*
*"How has this affected your day-to-day life?"* (this question often
brings out the other symptoms: poor concentration, loss of energy,
hopelessness, thoughts of harm)

*Past medical history/family history*
Depression, mania, DSH/suicide attempts, postnatal depression
Chronic disease, e.g. diabetes, COPD

*Drug history*
Benzodiazepines, sedatives, St John's wort, COCP
Previous treatments

**Social history**  Smoking, alcohol, recreational drugs
Work, home, relationships, family, finances
Children
Social support, housing

**Red flags**  *Always ask directly about suicide and suicidal intent*
Risk to self – DSH, suicide
Risk to others
Alternative diagnosis: hypothyroidism, anxiety, grief, PTSD, BPAD,
schizophrenia

**Examination**  Tearfulness, *"hearing voices?"*

## Interpersonal skills

**ICE**  Especially important to find out 'ICE' early on in consultation
Effect on life
Open questions, active listening, empathy

Important to involve patient in management plan
Is patient a carer?
Social isolation?

**For patient**
*"Depression affects 1 in 5 people at some point in their life"*
*"Depression affects different people differently, but generally it is when low mood affects your life and interferes with your everyday activities"*
*"Can be treated with a combination of self-help, talking therapies and medications if needed"*
*"Antidepressants take 2–4 weeks to work, and are not addictive"*
*"We normally advise taking antidepressants for 6 months after feeling better"*

## Management

**Investigations**
Consider bloods – TFTs (especially if no stressor)
Questionnaire: PHQ-9, HAD score

**Management**
*Conservative*
Support – family, friends, GP, counselling
Sleep hygiene, exercise, diet, stopping drugs/alcohol, watchful waiting
*Psychological intervention*
Low intensity: guided self-help, computerised CBT, group exercise programme
High intensity: CBT, interpersonal therapy
*Medical*
Antidepressants (SSRIs = first-line)
Sleeping tablets (for short-term use, e.g. 1–2 weeks; assess risk of overdose first)
*Social*
Benefits, sick note, social support, child protection issues

**Safety net**
Urgent referral if immediate risk to self/others
Refer if high risk/drug use/uncertain diagnosis and follow up in 1 week
Follow up in 2 weeks for most initial cases

## When to screen for depression

- Chronic disease, carer, life event (death, divorce, pregnancy...), drugs/alcohol, past history.

## Postnatal depression

- Affects up to 12% of women.
- Consider using Edinburgh Postnatal Depression Scale.

- Treat as for normal depression.
- Involve health visitor early.
- Lower threshold for non-drug treatments when patient is breastfeeding.
- Tricyclics better for breastfeeding women as more data and less secreted in breast milk.
- Be aware of child protection issues.
- If psychotic features refer to perinatal mental health team (possible puerperal psychosis).

# Summary of NICE (2009) and SIGN (2010) Guidelines on depression

*Always ask directly about suicide and suicidal intent*
If there is a risk:
- ask about social support
- inform how to get help depending on level of risk
- urgently refer/admit if immediate risk to self/others
- consider crisis resolution or home-treatment teams

### Treatment

Patient should be involved in assessing how well treatment is working.

Refer if not responding to therapy outlined below.

*General measures*
- Sleep hygiene:
  - regular sleeping/waking times
  - avoid excess alcohol, smoking, eating before sleep
  - environment conducive to sleep
- Exercise – also helps sleep
- Provide written information on depression
- Review – follow up in 2 weeks, contact patient if they do not attend

*Subthreshold or mild to moderate depression*
- Step 1: offer a low-intensity psychological intervention first
- Step 2: if this fails then offer antidepressant or high intensity psychological intervention
- Step 3: if decline therapies at step 2, consider counselling or short-term psychodynamic therapy

*Moderate to severe depression*
Antidepressant *and* high intensity psychological intervention (CBT or IPT).

Consider referral (for multidisciplinary care).

*Treating relapse*
- *Individual CBT* if significant PMH depression and failed antidepressant treatment.

- *Mindfulness-based cognitive therapy* if currently well with three episodes of past depression.
- May need to continue antidepressant, review after 2 years.
- Consider referral, e.g. for augmentation with lithium or antipsychotic.

### Low intensity psychological interventions

- *Individual guided self-help*
  - based on CBT principles
  - individual can be supported by trained professional
  - 6–8 sessions over 3 months
- *Computerised CBT*
  - Can be supported by trained professional
  - Over 3 months
- *Structured group exercise programme*
  - $3 \times 45$ min sessions/week over 3 months
- *Peer support group* if co-existing chronic disease

### High intensity psychological interventions

- *CBT*
- *Interpersonal therapy (IPT)*
- *Behavioural activation*
- *Behavioural couples therapy* if partner contributing to dynamics of depression
- *Group CBT* for people with chronic disease:
  - should be offered before individual CBT for people with chronic disease
  - groups of 8–10
  - over 3–4 months

### Antidepressants

Not routinely used for mild depression or persistent subthreshold symptoms that persist.

Continue for 6 months after remission (prevents relapse).

Consider increasing dose or changing drug if no improvement after 3–4 weeks.

Stop gradually over 4 weeks (less for fluoxetine, more for paroxetine and venlafaxine).

After starting antidepressant, review after:
- 2 weeks in most
- 1 week if increased suicide risk or age <30 years

Consider antidepressants if:
- moderate/severe depression
- subthreshold symptoms present for >2 years
- mild depression or persistent subthreshold symptoms unresponsive to above treatments
- mild depression complicating chronic disease

*SSRIs*
- First-line.
- Increased risk of GI bleeding: prescribe PPI if patient is elderly and taking aspirin/NSAID.
- Citalopram and sertraline have fewer drug interactions.
- Fluoxetine, fluvoxamine and paroxetine have more drug interactions.

*Specialist advice required for:*
- lithium augmentation, non-reversible MAOIs and combination antidepressants

## Antidepressants and co-existing chronic disease

No evidence that specific antidepressants good for specific conditions.

Beware of side-effects and interactions (e.g. SSRIs can exacerbate hyponatraemia, especially in elderly).

## If family/carers involved

Negotiate sharing of information.

Consider carer's assessment.

Provide written and verbal information on how to support patient.

**Electroconvulsive therapy** (ECT) is last resort treatment.

## Not recommended

Dosulepin.
St John's wort:
- lack of dose standardisation
- several interactions including with COCP, anticonvulsants and anticoagulants

# Anxiety

*Based on ICD-10 criteria and NICE Guidelines (2007)*

## Data gathering

| | |
|---|---|
| ***Symptoms*** | Clarify symptoms, e.g. apprehension, irritability, poor sleep, avoidance behaviour |

Clarify symptoms, e.g. apprehension, irritability, poor sleep, avoidance
   behaviour
When did symptoms first start?
Significant events – family, work, finances
*Panic disorder*
   Recurrent episodes, severe anxiety, unpredictable
*GAD*
   Symptoms present most of the time
*Phobia*
   In response to certain well defined situations that are not currently
      dangerous
*Others*
   Depression, hyperthyroidism

***Social history***  Caffeine, nicotine, alcohol, recreational drugs
Social support networks
Occupation

***Red flags***  Risk to self and/or others

***Examination***  Mental state
BP, pulse, heart

## Interpersonal skills

***ICE***  Effect on daily functioning and occupation
Depression can often co-exist

***For patient***  Inform patient that condition is treatable
Support groups and shared decision-making improves outcome

## Management

***Investigations***  Urine – catecholamines
Bloods – TFTs, glucose
ECG

*Management*   *Conservative*
          Exercise, relaxation techniques
          Avoid caffeine
     *Psychological*
          CBT for 1–4 months (longest lasting effect of all treatments – NICE)
          Self-help – computer-aided or bibliotherapy (CBT-based)
     *Medical*
          SSRI

*Safety net*   Refer to specialist if two interventions have no significant effect
     Monitor effect with self-complete questionnaires if possible

# SSRI

- For example, sertraline, for at least 6 months, then stop over 4–6 months.
- Warn the patient regarding initial worsening symptoms, delay in effect, and potential withdrawal symptoms if suddenly stopped.
- Can try another SSRI if first doesn't work after 12 weeks.

# Immediate management

*Based on NICE primary care guidelines*

- Benzodiazepines – for no longer than 2–4 weeks.
- Sedative antihistamines can also be used.
- Propranolol.

# Psychiatric risk assessment

For purposes of the CSA, if a risk assessment is required, then you should generally ask about three areas: risk of suicide, risk of self harm and risk of harming others. The questions can sometimes be difficult to ask in a real-life setting due to their directness – I find here that speaking slowly and with a caring/concerned tone helps enormously.

**In patients who present with low mood, always ask directly about suicide and suicidal intent.**

Remember, the risk of suicide is different to the risk of deliberate self-harm; e.g. a patient may have thoughts of harming themselves without suicidal ideation.

### 1. Risk of suicide

- Thoughts of harm to self.
- Previous suicidal attempts.

Here are some suggested phrases. First an opening question:

*"How do you feel about the future?"*

*"Have you had thoughts that life is not worth living?"* Note that this is an opening question and is not directly asking about suicidal ideation. It is possible for someone to have thoughts that life is not worth living but still not be actively suicidal. You must therefore ask a more direct question such as:

*"Have you had any thoughts of wanting to end your life?"*

*"Have you ever tried to end your life before?"*

---

You may need to work up to asking about suicidal ideas:
- *"How do you feel about the future?"*
- *"Have you had thoughts that life is not worth living?"*
- *"Do you have negative thoughts?"*
- *"Have you had any thoughts of wanting to end it all/end your life?"*
- *"Have you made any plans to end your life/kill yourself?"*

Suicide risk:
- *"Do you think you would try to end your life/kill yourself?"*
- *"What is stopping you?"*
- *"What will you do if you feel suicidal?"*

Risk of DSH:
- *"Have you had any thoughts of wanting to harm yourself?"*
- *"Have you ever hurt or harmed yourself before?"*

---

Risk to others:
- *"Have you had any thoughts or desires to hurt other people?"*
- *"Have you ever acted on these thoughts before?"*
- *"Have you had past involvement with the police or criminal justice/prison system?"*

If there is suicidal ideation, then further questions are required. An easy mnemonic is PALS:

**P**lans: does the patient have a plan to commit suicide vs. impulsive thoughts?
**A**ccess: is the plan available to the patient?
**L**ethality: how lethal is the method of proposed suicide?
**S**ocial support

## 2. Risk of deliberate self harm

- Thoughts of harming self.
- History of harming self.

*"Have you had any thoughts of wanting to harm yourself?"*

*"Have you ever hurt or harmed yourself before?"*

## 3. Risk to others

- Thoughts of harming others.
- History of harming others.
- Forensic history.

*"Have you had any thoughts or desires to hurt other people?"*

*"Have you ever acted on these thoughts before?"*

*"Have you had past involvement with the police or criminal justice/prison system?"*

Also ask about alcohol, recreational drugs, and past psychiatric history.

## If there is a risk:

- ask about social support
- inform how to get help depending on level of risk
- urgently refer/admit if immediate risk to self/others
- consider crisis resolution or home-treatment teams

# Recent non-accidental overdose

## Data gathering

*History*
    *"Tell me how it happened?"*
    Number of tablets taken, what dose of what medication
    ?Taken all at once or over a period of time (clarify time), ?with alcohol
    *"Did you make any plans so you wouldn't be found?"*
    *"Did you write a suicide note or will?"*
    *"How long have you been feeling this way for?"*
    Motivation
      *"Why did you do it?"*
      *"Was there anything that happened that made you do it?"*
      *"Was this something you planned to do?"*
      *"How did you feel:*
- *before you did it?"*
- *when you were doing it?"*

    Risk to self
      Impulsive vs. premeditated
      Cry for help vs. serious intent
      *"How do you feel about it now?"*
      *"Do you still think of harming yourself?"*
      *"What is stopping you from harming yourself now?"*
      *"What will you do if you feel this way again?"*
      *"Have you ever tried to harm or kill yourself before?"*
    Psychiatric history
      History of mental illness – depression, schizophrenia
      Previous attempts at suicide/self harm

*Social history*
    Social support network – *"Is there anyone you can turn to for support?"*
    Work, home, relationships, finances
    Smoking, alcohol, recreational drugs
    Child protection issues

*Red flags*
    Risk of harm to self/others, psychiatric illness
    Drug abuse, poor social support
    Immediate risk of overdose

*Examination*
    Mental state

## Interpersonal skills

*ICE*    Expectations, e.g. sick note, referral, support group

## Management

*Investigations*    Risk assessment

*Management*    Refer if high risk
Support groups – AA, substance misuse

*Safety net*    Review in 1 week if low risk and no medical problems
"*What do you feel needs to happen for you to feel in control of your life again?*"
"*What would you do if you felt this way again?*"

# Alcoholism

## Data gathering

**History**   Number of units per week
Binge vs. daily
Social vs. alone
*CAGE*
   Need to **C**ut down?
   **A**nnoyed at criticism to cut down?
   **G**uilty about drinking?
   **E**ye opener – need an early morning drink?

**Social history**   Driving

**Red flags**   Memory, blackouts, functioning, injuries
Depression, stress, suicide risk
Delirium tremens, haematemesis

**Examination**   BP, weight
Tremor, speech
Hands, pulse, jaundice, anaemia, heart, abdomen
Neuropathy, encephalopathy

## Interpersonal skills

**ICE**   Effect on life
Explore ideas of why patient drinks excessively, e.g. stress at home or at
   work, issues from childhood, social environment

**For patient**   Explain risks of alcohol (see below)

## Management

**Investigations**   Bloods – FBC (macrocytosis), LFT, gamma-GT
Urine – toxicology screen

**Management**   *Conservative*
   Emphasise stopping drinking is patient's responsibility
   Alcohol diary, Alcoholics Anonymous, support to patient and family
   Inform DVLA
*Medical*
   Vitamin B and C
   Consider detoxification (see below)

*Other*
Treat depression

*Safety net*    Regular review
Admit delirium tremens, haematemesis, pancreatitis

# Alcohol detoxification

- Motivation to stop – emphasise patient is responsible for detox success.
- Detox in community over 1 week with chlordiazepoxide, daily dispensing from pharmacy.
- Refer for detox if:
  - delirium tremens/seizures
  - drug user
  - lack of social support

---

**Units**

1 unit = $\frac{1}{2}$ pint beer, 25 ml spirits, 125 ml wine

Bottle of wine = 9 units

Recommended intake: men <3–4 units per day, women <2–3 units per day; avoid alcohol for 2–3 days after a heavy drinking session

---

# Risks of alcohol

- *"It affects every organ in body"*.
- Injuries.
- Erectile dysfunction, infertility.
- Brain damage, depression.
- Obesity, diabetes, heart disease.
- Liver damage.
- Cancer: breast, mouth, oesophagus, liver.

# Delirium tremens

- Onset is 2–3 days after patient stops drinking.
- Fever, tachycardia, tachypnoea, high BP, visual hallucinations, tremor, confusion, fits.

# Insomnia and sleep disorders

## Data gathering

*Time course*   Short-term (<4 weeks) vs. long-term (>4 weeks)
Past-history of insomnia
Every day vs. occasionally
Difficulty falling asleep vs. interrupted sleep vs. early morning waking
Sleeping routine – when go to bed/wake up? Sleep during day?

*Ideas*   "*Do you have any idea why you have difficulty sleeping?*"
- Stressor, e.g. family, at work, finances, stressful event
- Symptom, e.g. cough, pain, apnoea, nocturia
- Stimulants, e.g. caffeine

Previous treatments tried

*Social history*   Home, work, relationships, finances
Smoking, alcohol, recreational drugs, caffeine

*Red flags*   Depression and anxiety screen
Drug abuse, alcoholism
Hypothyroidism
Hyperthyroidism

*Examination*

## Interpersonal skills

*ICE*   Open questions at the beginning followed by listening will often give you the context for insomnia without you having to ask all the specifics
Effect on life, e.g. problems during the day concentrating, driving
Important to establish early on what patient wants from doctor and use this to guide management

## Management

*Investigations*   Often none required, TFTs
Investigations directed by cause

*Management*   Treat cause
*Conservative*
Sleep hygiene (see **Tired all the time**)
Avoid caffeine and alcohol

Symptom diary can be helpful

*Psychological*

CBT is first-line for insomnia >4 weeks duration

*Medical*

Sedative medications (e.g. zopiclone, temazepam)

- generally indicated only for short-term insomnia (<4 weeks)
- usually only prescribe for 1–2 weeks at a time
- explain risks:
    - long term: addiction, tolerance, cognitive impairment, ataxia
    - short term: hangover effects, daytime drowsiness and impaired judgement

***Safety net*** Review as appropriate

[**Note**] whilst alcohol is a sedative, it also causes disrupted sleep patterns.

# Eating disorders

*Based on NICE Guidelines (2004)*

## Data gathering

**Screening**  *"Do you think you have an eating problem?"*
*"Do you worry excessively about your weight?"*
*Symptoms*
Bingeing, purging, laxatives
Restriction diet, exercise
Body image, fear fatness
Periods, thyroid, GIT
*Past medical history*
Depression, anxiety, other psychiatric history

**Social history**  Work, home, relationships

**Red flags**  BMI <60% of normal
Poor social support, co-morbidities (psychiatric/physical), pregnancy
Suicide risk

**Examination**  Weight, BMI, pulse, BP
Mental state

## Interpersonal skills

**ICE**  Importance of gaining rapport and patient's trust
Empathy, non-judgemental attitude
Issues of confidentiality if patient is a child

## Management

**Investigations**  U&Es, DEXA

**Management**  Support patient, reassure that assistance is available
*Conservative*
Food diary
Self help programme
Family therapies for children/adolescents
Support groups
*Psychological*
CBT – refer early

*Medical*
SSRI – e.g. fluoxetine 60 mg daily (higher dose than for depression)

***Safety net*** Monitor extensively if type I diabetes or pregnant
Admit if weight <60% of normal or risk of suicide or medical complications

*"Laxative abuse does not greatly reduce calorie absorption"*.

After vomiting:
- avoid brushing
- rinse with non-acid mouthwash

# Opiate addiction

## Data gathering

*History*   Establish patient's agenda, e.g.:
- wanting opiates to prevent withdrawal
- wanting help for stabilisation/detoxification
- other, e.g. finances, housing

Ever injected drugs? Shared needles? Hepatitis B?

*Collateral history*
   From psychiatrist, drug treatment centre, another GP

*Social history*   Housing, finances
Smoking, alcohol, recreational drugs

*Red flags*   Pregnancy, child protection issues

*Examination*   Pulse, BP
Injection sites, infection/sepsis, opiate withdrawal

## Interpersonal skills

*ICE*   Reassure patient either you and/or a specialist centre will help support him
Effectively deal with aggression or demanding patient without provoking
   patient

## Management

*Investigations*   Urine – drugs screen
Bloods – Hep B and C, HIV

*Management*   Smoking is safer than injection
*Conservative*
   Support groups
   Needle exchange programmes, don't share needles, safe needle disposal
   Hepatitis B immunisation
*Medical*
   Methadone or buprenophine stabilisation/detoxification
   As a general rule do not prescribe opiates on first encounter
   Treat withdrawal symptoms as needed, e.g. propranolol, loperamide
*Social*
   Benefits, accommodation, occupation, sick notes

*Safety net*    Refer if complex case or depending on local service agreements

# Opiate withdrawal

*Symptoms*: abdominal pain, agitation, diarrhoea, dilated pupils, rhinorrhoea, sweating, vomiting.

Remember patients cannot die from withdrawal symptoms (although they may feel they will) but they can die from methadone/opiate overdose.

# Cannabis abuse

## Data gathering

*History*    How often? Method (smoked, eaten)? Setting?
Why started?
Any problems encountered?
*Screen for harmful effects*
   See below
*Past medical history*
   Cardiovascular disease
   Psychiatric history

*Social history*    Occupation, use of heavy machinery, driving
Smoking, alcohol, other recreational drugs, intravenous drug use

*Red flags*    Dependence, schizophrenia

*Examination*    Weight, BP, pulse

## Interpersonal skills

*ICE*    Effect on life, relationships, occupation
Screen for anxiety and depression
Some heavy users may have financial difficulties

*To patient*    Explain potential harmful effects of use (see below)

## Management

*Investigations*    Consider urine toxicology screen

*Management*    Advise on stopping
Advise on harmful effects, written information
Advise regarding law:
- illegal
- currently a Class B drug

*Safety net*    Review social and financial support

# Harmful effects of cannabis

- Cognition: memory loss, irritability.
- Respiratory: cough, wheeze, recurrent respiratory infection.
- Schizophrenia: delusions, hallucinations, delusions of thought control.
- Problems with fertility.
- Dependence, tolerance.

# Post-traumatic stress disorder

*Based on NICE Guidelines (2005)*

## Data gathering

**History**   PTSD occurs after exceptionally threatening event, e.g. rape, assault, torture, road traffic accident (i.e. not after divorce, failing exams or loss of job)

Three main features:
1. flashbacks, nightmares – often vivid
2. avoidance behaviour – avoid similar situations
3. emotional numbing or hyper-arousal

Also irritability, anger

**Social history**   Occupation (higher incidence in those working for the military, police, and emergency services)

Alcohol, recreational drugs

**Red flags**   Risk of suicide and deliberate self harm

Risk of harming others

**Examination**   Mental state

## Interpersonal skills

**ICE**   Depression screen, may experience grief, effect on life

Consider screening for PTSD in those at high risk

## Management

**Investigations**

**Management**   If <4 weeks since event, manage with watchful waiting (unless very severe symptoms)

*Conservative*

Encourage family involvement if possible

Support groups

Treat any drug abuse before treating PTSD

*Psychological*

Trauma-focused CBT

Eye movement desensitisation and reprocessing

*Medical*

    Drug treatment not first line, generally to be initiated by specialist
      e.g. paroxetine, mirtazepine

    Short-term sedatives may be required for sleep disturbance

**Safety net**   Regular review for patient support

Generally needs referral for specialist assessment and treatment

Beware red flags

# Appendix 1 – Influenza vaccination

## Influenza vaccine

Yearly to:

- >65s
- chronic disease: respiratory (including asthma on inhaled steroids), CHD, chronic renal failure, diabetes
- immunosuppressed: e.g. asplenia
- nursing home residents and carers
- healthcare professionals

# Appendix 2 – History taking

## Cardiovascular history

- Chest pain
- SOB – exertion, orthopnoea, PND
- Palpitations
- Syncope, pre-syncope
- Ankle oedema

*Cardiovascular risk factors:*
- modifiable: smoking, hypertension, raised cholesterol
- non-modifiable: male, increasing age, South Asian origin, family history or past medical history of CVD, CKD, DM, PVD

Ask about respiratory symptoms.

## Respiratory history

- Cough
- Shortness of breath
- Wheeze
- Sputum/haemoptysis
- Chest pain

## Gastro-intestinal history

- Abdominal pain
- Nausea, vomiting, diarrhoea
- Weight loss, appetite, diet
- Bowel habit, bleeding
- Consider ectopic in all female patients with abdominal pains

Ask about GU symptoms

## Genito-urinary history

*Irritative*: dysuria, urgency, frequency, incontinence (stress vs. urge)
*Obstructive*: hesitancy, dribbling/poor stream, nocturia
Haematuria
Testicular pain/swelling
Vaginal discharge (women)

Obstetric and gynaecology history (women)
Sexual history
Ask about GI symptoms

# Pain history

**S**ite
**O**nset
**C**haracter
**R**adiation
**A**lleviating factors
**T**ime course
**E**xacerbating factors
**S**igns and symptoms associated

*"Have you ever had this before?"*
*"Have you tried anything to help the pain? (any medication?)"*
ICE

# Abdominal pain history

- Relationship to food
- Could patient be pregnant? – LMP, unprotected sexual intercourse, etc.
- GI symptoms
- GU symptoms

+/– examining hernial orifices, external genitalia, PR, bimanual
+/– urine dip/MSU

Diagnoses – DKA, glaucoma, migraine

# Gynaecology history

Most important are:
- pregnancy (including ectopic)
- STI risk
- periods – LMP, how many days between periods (most and fewest days), how many days bleeding
- PCB, IMB, dyspareunia
- contraception
- last smear

Ask yourself: could patient be pregnant? e.g. feeling faint, vomiting, weight gain.

# Obstetric history

- Pregnancies
- Miscarriage
- Termination of pregnancy
- Caesarean sections
- Consider postnatal depression for obstetric cases

# Sexual history

- Ascertain risk of pregnancy or STI
- Sexually active? With who? Regular partner?
- Use condom? Contraception?
- Any accidents? Missed pill?
- Are you worried about STI?
- Pain? Discharge?
- PCB
- Does partner have any symptoms?
- LMP?

# Appendix 3 – Suggested phrases during a consultation

As stated throughout the book, use the phrases that you feel comfortable with and that fit within your consultation style. If you have any suggestions, please let me know!

| | |
|---|---|
| **Open questions** | *"What brings you here today?"*<br>*"Can you tell me more about 'X'?"*<br>*"How did it all begin?"* |
| **Presenting complaint** | *"What do you mean by 'X'?"*<br>*"Have you ever had this before?"*<br>*"Have you already tried anything?"*<br>*"Was there anything in particular that made you come to see a doctor now (rather than before)?"* |
| **Social history** | *"Who lives at home?"*<br>*"How are things at work? Outside work?"*<br>*"Has anything happened at home/work?"* |
| **ICE and effect on daily life** | *"Do you have any idea what is causing this?"*<br>*"Is there anything in particular that you are concerned about?"*<br>*"Is there anything in particular you were hoping I could do for you today?"*<br>*"How does this affect your day-to-day life?"*<br>*"Does it stop you from doing anything?"*<br>*"How are you coping with it all?"* |
| **Empathy statements** | *"That must be very difficult for you..."*<br>*"Sounds like you've been through a lot..."*<br>*"I'm so sorry to hear that..."*<br>*"I understand that must be quite annoying for you..."* |
| **Picking up cues** | Non-verbal<br>    *"How are you feeling?"*<br>    *"How do you feel about what's been said so far?"*<br>Verbal<br>    *"You mentioned that you look after your grandmother..."* |
| **Abusive patients** | *"I am trying to listen to you but can't whilst you are using such bad language"*<br>*"Maybe it would be better to do this at another time when you are less offensive"*<br>An effective phrase in real life is *"Do you realise that you are shouting?"* |

## General pointers to build rapport

*Non-verbal:*      eye contact, smile

*Verbal*:      speak clearly, soft tone of voice, avoid monotonous tone/vary pitch of voice

*Active listening:*   gently nodding head, open body language, non-judgemental

## Difficult, direct or intrusive questions and consultations

Use soft and caring tone with a slow and almost hesitant pace. It's not only what you say, but how you say it.

# Summary of consultation structure

## The five key steps

1. Initial open question
2. Targeted history with red flags
3. Ideas, concerns, expectations (ICE) and effect on day-to-day life
4. Explain diagnosis and shared management plan
5. Safety net/arrange follow up

## Data gathering

| | |
|---|---|
| *Introduction* | Open question(s) |
| | "*What brings you here today?*" |
| | "*Can you tell me more about 'X'?*" |
| | "*How did it all begin?*" |
| *Targeted history* | Presenting complaint |
| | "*What do you mean by 'X'?*" |
| | "*Have you ever had this before?*" |
| | "*Have you already tried anything?*" |
| | "*Was there anything in particular that made you come to see a doctor now (rather than before)?*" |
| | Past medical history |
| | Family history |
| | Drug history |
| | Drug concordance, OTC/herbal remedies |
| *Social history* | Home, job, relationships |
| | "*Who lives at home?*" |
| | "*How are things at work? Outside work?*" |
| | "*Has anything happened at home/work?*" |
| | Smoking, alcohol, drugs |
| *Red flags* | e.g. bleeding, pain, weight loss |
| | Examination if required |
| *Targeted examination* | If required |

## Interpersonal skills

| | |
|---|---|
| *ICE and effect on daily life* | "*Do you have any idea what is causing this?*" |
| | "*Is there anything in particular that you are concerned about?*" |
| | "*Is there anything in particular you were hoping I could do for you today?*" |
| | "*How does this affect your day-to-day life?*" and/or "*Does it stop you from doing anything?*" |
| | "*How are you coping with it all?*" |
| | Summarise |
| *For patient* | Explain diagnosis |

## Management

| | |
|---|---|
| *Suggested investigations* | Urine, bloods, imaging if required |
| *Management options* | Conservative, medical, surgical |
| | Lifestyle, social |
| *Safety net* | Arrange follow up |
| | Consider referral (e.g. if red flags) |